Calisthenics

Flexibility for Bodyweight Training Guide

(The True Bodyweight Training Guide Your Body Deserves)

Anthony Mitchell

Published By **Tyson Maxwell**

Anthony Mitchell

All Rights Reserved

Calisthenics: Flexibility for Bodyweight Training Guide (The True Bodyweight Training Guide Your Body Deserves)

ISBN   978-1-998038-60-2

Legal & Disclaimer

Table Of Contents

Chapter 1: What Is Calisthenics

Calisthenics refers to an workout that can be done with no equipment and instead, it's performed with the help of your body to increase muscles. They are typically performed in a synchronized manner through using gross motor abilities. One of the advantages of calisthenics is that it does not have to venture out to buy expensive equipment. You don't need an exercise membership, you don't require a coach or buy a lot of complex exercises videos.

What you must perform is to use your body to assist you in losing pounds and gain muscles. In addition to not spending hundreds of dollars for products you'll probably not need in the future, when you use your body for calisthenics, the focus is on controlling the body rather than focusing on how much weight you could take on. Imagine the situation in this manner. If you train to lift, you will improve your lifting skills since we have learned that practicing is the key to perfection, however when you're practicing control of the body then that's the thing you'll become proficient in.

One of the benefits of using calisthenics in place of weightlifting is that, unlike weightlifting, calisthenics encourages the growth of muscles that are lean, whereas weightlifting gives you an increase in bulk. It means calisthenics could be enjoyed by both males as well as women, without having to be concerned about getting too heavy.

Of course, there's no problem with lifting weights If this is something you're looking to accomplish. I am all for it, however since you're studying this book, I'm going to assume that weight lifting isn't suitable for you.

If you're looking to get healthier and more lean, then calisthenics could be for you however if you're looking to build up your strength, the workouts which I'll show you in this guide aren't beneficial for your needs. But If you are looking to reduce weight and increase muscles that are lean, then you'll be awed by what calisthenics could do to help you.

The calisthenics exercise can be done by anybody of any level of fitness. If you've had no exercise in your entire life, it is possible to do calisthenics. There is no need to fret about staying on top of the lady who is dancing on the screen, as the time you buy an aerobics DVD. You can do it at your own speed therefore if it takes some time to complete 10 repetitions, it's acceptable.

The very first thing you must do with regards to calisthenics is set goals. If you've been unable to exercise, however you are hoping complete 100 reps on an exercise. It's not necessary to stress about 100 reps the first day of working on your goal for the future. To achieve your goal for the short term it could be that you complete 5 repetitions of the particular workout every day over the course of one week. In the following week, it could be that you'll be able to do 7 reps and then 10 reps in the week following and on.

For each of the exercises I offer the reader in this book, you'll need be able to establish goals that you can reach. The final chapter in this book, I'm going to set the opportunity to set a 21-day goal for you to help you get towards more reps for each exercise. However, if you find this challenge not working for you, then make your own using this guidelines.

Once you've decided on the number of reps you would like to perform for each workout, it is important to consider the bigger image. What is the reason you are doing calisthenics? Do you wish to lose pounds? What amount of weight do you wish to shed? Are you looking to develop strong muscles? How strong would you like to become?

Which other activities are you planning to incorporate into your training routine? What's great of calisthenics is you are able to do 10 reps here, and 5 reps in the next when you've got some time however, you'll also need to incorporate an aerobic workout in addition to your calisthenics.

It is not my intention to discuss this as I prefer to be focusing on calisthenics however, if you're trying to lose weight, you'll need more to accomplish than increase the amount of the lean mass of your muscles. Naturally, that's likely to assist you in losing pounds, but there's more involved than that.

It is also important to select an aerobic workout that you could do handful of times each week you are interested in. This is essential and is the same for calisthenics as well. If you aren't enjoying exercising, you're probably unlikely to commit to it. If you don't commit to the program, you'll never be able to see the results you desire. This is because, instead of enjoying your work out, it will make you dread the task every single day. You will begin to be feeling like it's an obligation you are required to complete and would rather not do. If you do not want to complete it, you're likely to come up with reasons not to take on the task.

Decide on an aerobic activity that you enjoy and one you can keep doing. Even if you need to change things up each day, make sure to be sure to keep it exciting and make sure that you're enjoying yourself.

Chapter 2: Nutrition

It is impossible to lose weight or be healthy weight if your don't modify the way you're eating. The importance of nutrition is the same as and as exercise in relation to losing weight. The body needs adequate fuel in order to need it to function properly which is why the nutrition and the hydration factor in.

I'm an avid proponent of eating clean. Personally, I am of the opinion that if a food item is manufactured in a laboratory, the food should not go in the body. There is no way to guarantee that if you put your body in contact with an array of chemicals they will work properly.

This is why I want to discuss processed foods. It's time to start by looking at all the food products that are labelled as 'low fat' , no sugar as well as other foods that are diet-friendly. It is true that lower fat and low fat, or low fat food items are still containing the same amount of sugar, or greater than the original food as sugar is fat free. If you are looking for the sugar free food options, these can be just as bad for your health because instead of containing sugar, they replace sugar with sweet chemical.

Perhaps you are thinking that sugar is a natural ingredient. Sugar cane is what you purchase in the grocery store, and the stuff you in your food are refined sugar. White flour that is used in food items has been bleached and deprives of all its nutritional value. Foods like Cheetos are just scientific tests.

I could go on about how harmful the food you eat throughout the day, but I don't. I want you to know how it impacts the body. I strongly suggest you go to the film FEDUP in order to fully understand the harm you're inflicting on your body taking these foods.

Certain people are able to eliminate these meals in a hurry, but I would suggest doing gradually to ensure that you don't make your body go through withdrawals. The sugar present in these meals triggers your brain to experience a an identical reaction to cocaine. This is extremely addictive, as well as, like cocaine, it can make your body suffer symptoms when you don't provide the addict with. It is possible to feel unwell in your first week free of refined sugar. You might feel feeling lightheaded and exhausted as good. It's normal, and should be something you plan for.

After you have figured out the foods you shouldn't eat, there is a need to know about what foods to be eating. Organic fruits, vegetables meat, dairy and other foods are what you have to center your eating habits around. Instead of sodas be sure you're drinking enough fluids. It is essential to drink enough water to allow your body to shed excess fat, and also if you would like to build muscle.

Dairy products need some explanation as fruits, vegetables as well as meat. It is because many the majority of people are confused as to the best dairy products to consume. People drink skim milk, indulge in vegetable oil spreads and low fat cheeses, thinking they're doing themselves an favor. The reality is that you're causing damage to your body taking this route.

It is essential to drink full milk, use real butter and eat real cheese. There is no need for American Cheese slices, these aren't really cheese but cheese products and if you search for a video on YouTube explaining how the cheese makes its way through the process, you'll not touch it ever once more. The reason why you're eating them is because they're as close to their original state as is possible which is exactly what you are aiming at.

It is important to concentrate on having food items that are in their most natural conditions as you can. It doesn't mean everything you eat needs to be prepared in raw form, as you can cook them, however when eating fruits or vegetables it's better to consume as much in the raw state as possible.

It is true that you may not be able go 100 % without any processed food however a good guideline to live to is that it's acceptable to consume it so you can eat it as long as there are three ingredients or less, and you are aware of what the ingredients include. (I have seen chocolate bars that look like these)

When you're eating like this, you're likely have to consume a A LOT. Foods you'll take in do not include as much calories as you're used to. One benefit of taking the plunge into this new lifestyle is that you won't ever be thirsty.

Take a look at this. In terms of the calories that you get from the regular size snickers bars it is possible to eat two half and a quarter bananas. The best part about this is that you're not likely to have to eat two and half bananas to snack on, which will mean that you're getting rid of calories and also giving your body what nutrients is required.

In relation to your meals, you'll need ensure that you're getting 14g of fiber every 1,000 calories you're eating every day. That's 2 cups of fruits, 2.5 cups of vegetables and the protein content is 46 grams for women and 56 grams for males.

It is also important to ensure you're taking in enough complex carbohydrates, starchy carbs as well as healthy fats. If you aren't getting these nutrients, you'll begin suffer from fatigue and feel downright sick. Avocados are an excellent option to obtain the nutritious fats you requlre, potatoes provide you with simple carbohydrates, and complex carbs are found in beans and whole grains. They also include seeds, nuts and fruits and veggies.

It is recommended to drink a minimum of 8 glasses of fluids per daily. Every morning, when you get up, instead of heading straight to the cafe, take the glass of water you have then squeeze out the juice of one lemon in it. It will provide your metabolism with an increase as you get up, and it helps you to burn more calories throughout your whole day.

If you feel thirsty, sip one glass of water before eating. Many times, people mistake their thirst with hunger which causes them to consume more food. If you start drinking the fluids your body needs, you'll notice that it's much simpler to shed the excess pounds.

Chapter 3: Exercises

The time has come to learn the basic calisthenics principles. In this chapter, I will cover the different exercises are available to you. I'll also give you the link to a YouTube video that will allow you to understand how this exercise performed.

Chest dip– This workout will focus on the chest area and is one of the exercises that require that you have more than your body. For this workout, you will require two bars that are parallel to each other. Most times, they are available in a park or fitness center. There are many who will say that the exercise will work your triceps and biceps however this isn't the case. The focus of this exercise is the chest, and very minimal work performed through the triceps and biceps. This is an instructional video on how this can be done.

https://www.youtube.com/watch?v=tUOETUfcCEI

The Pushups are one of the most fundamental workouts, however it's an entire body workout. They are a great way to build the upper part of your body, and assist in strengthening the muscles of the muscle groups in the center. They work a variety of muscle groups in the same workout. This includes arms, the chest and neck muscles, as well as triceps. shoulder and back. They help promote good posture as well as provide stability to the body. The pushups can also improve endurance and boost overall fitness. That is why military personnel utilize pushups as a part of their workout routine. They are incredibly simple to master and there are many kinds of pushups that target specific muscle groups. This video will teach you how to perform a simple pushup that is suitable for novices and various variations too.

https://www.youtube.com/watch?v=NECcLiefy0M

Squats- This workout will strengthen the entire leg as well as the lower back. This is an all-in one workout that targets your legs. You can sense every aspect of your legs working. This is an excellent video that demonstrates how to squat correctly.

https://www.youtube.com/watch?v=rXJzj9K3sxU

Lunges- This activity stimulates the lower body, and provides a good workout for your legs. The lunges work on the hip muscles as well as the muscles of the lower legs and abdominal muscles. This exercise is great for strengthening your core muscles and to focus on posture, too. Below is a fantastic video to master the art of the proper lunge.

https://www.youtube.com/watch?v=vNgs9ag uMw4

The crunches exercise can assist you in strengthening your core muscles by exercising the abdominal muscles. Additionally, it will help you concentrate on controlling the body, as it is crucial to control all of your movements when the crunches are being performed. Below is a video showing precisely how to do this.

https://www.youtube.com/watch?v=73CmRb QKDjY

Bench dips- This workout can be used to strengthen the triceps muscles. It is located at the top part of the arm. Many women struggle with the arm area that is that are gaining fat. However, with this workout you will burn the fat as well as build up the muscle mass that is lean. This video describes how you can do it.

https://www.youtube.com/watch?v=dl8_opV0A0Y

Scissor kicks - This exercise is excellent to work the muscles deep in your hips. However, it can also aid in strengthening abdominals and the legs. It's a basic exercise that has become very well-known due to this. Find this link for an instructional video on how to perform this workout.

https://www.youtube.com/watch?v=nWKTmFv76I8

Burpees- This type of exercise can be a little more difficult than other exercises have been taught to us so far. It is due to the fact that it is a Burpee is a total body workout that involves each muscle in the body. It's also known by the name of squat thrust, and the theory is that it was invented by a person named Burpee who was in a prison without fitness equipment. The following video will explain the process.

https://www.youtube.com/watch?v=B3pfaQ2sDPA

Knee High- A knee high will concentrate the abdominal muscles in your lower back more so than crunches. If you lift your knee, you're battling gravity. You are activating your abdominal muscles in the lower part of your body and each time you do it, you'll notice more and the muscles are burning. Below is a fantastic video for you to learn how to perform these exercises correctly.

https://www.youtube.com/watch?v=bZUfaLxJ36M

Forearm Planks- This exercise can help strengthen every muscle on the body's front that includes your arms, legs and lower back. It also strengthens your glutes, thighs and the core. It has been shown to improve a more positive attitude. Some people believe this appears to be a simple exercise, however when practicing it, you'll realize that your muscles are engaged, and this isn't as easy as it appears. This is an instructional video that will show you the correct way to complete this workout in a proper manner.

https://www.youtube.com/watch?v=xFGXIM oArw4

Calf raises- This workout concentrates on the calf. But it can help increase the strength of the ankle and knee too. This is a simple move that lots of individuals love because it provides those sexy calves and requires little effort. Below is the video that explains how you can perform this workout.

https://www.youtube.com/watch?v=-M4-G8p8fmc

Side torso lift- This exercise can assist in the development of muscles and also work on the shoulders and lower back in addition. It will involve the entire body when performing this workout. Below is a video that will show you the best way to complete this workout.

https://www.youtube.com/watch?v=eRu1Ol
m431g

These are the 12 best exercises you could begin by doing and you are able to add additional exercises into your regimen when you get more healthy. After we've learned about these exercises, which are the muscles that they focus on and, hopefully, you've seen all the videos to be sure that you're performing the exercises correctly, you can take on the 21-day test.

Chapter 4: 21 Day Challenge

Once you have a good understanding about calisthenics, nutrition, and the workouts you'll performing, it's the time to get ready for the calisthenics 21-day exercise challenge. This chapter we're going to review each day for the next 21 days in detail which exercises to perform along with the number of repetitions you must complete.

In this period you'll notice you're becoming more and better with these workouts, and you feel better than ever before ever felt before in your experience. Additionally, you will shed weight. That is exactly what this exercise is about!

Keep in mind that you are focused on eating a healthy diet and drinking plenty of water throughout the day. If you don't do this, you will see your results fall and you'll become frustrated. Be aware that it is only three weeks of your time and the results are worthy of the time and effort you'll be required to invest in it.

Day 1-

20 minutes of walking

Interval-

5 pushups

15 crunches

10 Squats

Three times. Repeat. As you begin to start out, you are able to do as many intervals as you're able to. If you're at intermediate every interval should last about 2 minutes. If you're at an advanced level, you'll need to complete one session for 60 seconds.

Day 2-

Cardio: Your cardio today is likely to differ from the norm. While you're working out, be sure you're not taking a break. To perform your workout, you'll take the following steps:

Jumping jacks for 10 second and knee the highs to 20 second. Jumping the jacks for 30 seconds knee highs lasting 40 seconds, jump at 50 second jacks and knee highs up to 60 seconds, jump the jacks to 50 seconds, the knees are elevated for 40 seconds and jumping jacks up to 30 seconds and knee highs for 20 seconds, and then jumping jacks every 10 seconds.

It's only six minutes of workout, so keep in the direction you want to go and you'll succeed in finishing.

Interval-

30 seconds forearm plank

5 burpees

Three times during your day.

Day 3-

Cardio Aim for 60 minutes of exercise

Interval-

5 chest dips

5 pushups

3 Squats

The interval will be done five times. If you're a beginner and want to learn, go as long as you want. Intermediates should not take more than 2 minutes while advanced will take less than a minute each time.

Day 4-

Cardio: 15 minutes jogging

Interval 1-

16 jumping jacks

6 crunches

5 side torso raises

Interval 2-

14 jumping jacks

4 crunches

6 side torso raises

Interval 3-

12 jumping jacks

6 crunches

7 side torso raises

Interval 4-

10 jumping jacks

4 crunches

8 side torso raises

Interval 5-

8 jumping jacks

6 crunches

9 side torso raises

Day 5-

Exercise- Walk for 20 minutes

Interval-

10 Squats

Ten pushups

10 burpees

10 lunges

Repeat 3 times.

Day 6-

Cardio- Jog for 30 minutes

Interval-

5 burpees

5 crunches

5 scissor kicks

5 lunges

Repeat 5 times.

Day 7-

Exercise- Walk for about 60 minutes

Interval-

The knees are elevated for 60 seconds.

5 pushups

10 lunges

12 crunches

12 Squats

12 scissor kicks

Day 8-

Exercise - Walk for 20 minutes, run 10 minutes, then run for 5 minutes

Interval-

10 second sprints

4 pushups

4 Squats

20 second sprints

4 pushups

6 Squats

30 second sprints

8 pushups

10 Squats

20 second sprints

4 pushups

6 Squats

10 second sprints

2 pushups

4 Squats

Day 9-

Exercise - 30 minutes walk

No interval

Day 10-

Cardio- 30 minutes of jogging then 30 second sprints followed by a walk for 30 seconds. Sprint 5 times and repeat.

Interval-

12 crunches

14 Squats

4 pushups

10 crunches

16 Squats

6 pushups

8 crunches

14 Squats

4 pushups

6 crunches

16 Squats

6 pushups

Day 11-

Cardio - 30 minutes of walking

Interval-

60 second forearm planek

10 side torso raises

60 second plank forearm

10 side torso raises

Day 12-

Walking 1 mile for cardio

Interval-

10 jumping jacks

Ten pushups

10 burpees

Pause for 10 seconds, then repeat the interval five times.

Day 13-

Exercise Walk 1 mile, accompanied by two pounds of weight added.

Interval-

6 lunges

8 Squats

6 pushups

Repeat this interval 4 times

Day 14-

Cardio- Run 1 mile

Interval-

Ten pushups

20 crunches

Repeat the interval four times

Day 15-

Cardio- Jog 2 miles

Interval-

12 crunches

6 pushups

6 burpees

10 calf raises

Repeat four times

Day 16-

Cardio- Jog 1 mile

Interval- no interval

Day 17-

Interval-

6 Squats

6 crunches

4 pushups

6 burpees

Repeat 5 times.

Day 18-

Exercise - Walk for 1 mile

15 jumping jacks

15 push-ups

15 lunges

10 burpees

15 chest dips

15 scissor kicks

15 knee highs

15 side torso raises

60 second forearm plank

Day 19-

Exercise - Run 2 miles

Interval-

15 jumping jacks

15 pushups

15 lunges

Repeat 3 times.

Day 20-

Cardio- Jog for 2 miles

Interval-

15 lunges

15 crunches

15 calf raises

15 scissor kicks

Repeat the interval four times

Day 21-

Fitness - 1 hour run

Interval-

16 scissor kicks

6 pushups

12 lunges

Repeat 5 times.

It's the 21-day calisthenics exercise goal. If you've reached this point, you'll look back on it with joy. When you turn 21 on the 21st day, you're likely to be a totally different person than the day before and that's something you should feel proud of.

While exercising, be sure you drink sufficient fluids. If it's hot out, you should be mindful about how much the water you consume. If the weather isn't allowing the outside to be enjoyable, it's okay to use a different type of cardio workout, provided you do it for exactly the same duration that you need during the time of day.

It is evident that there aren't any days in this challenge of 21 days, however this doesn't mean you shouldn't take day off. If you're a novice and want to get started, I recommend include 8 days in the challenge to ensure that your body capable of resting. In those days, you'll be doing no cardio, or do intervals. Instead, give your body time to relax and recuperate.

The muscles you work with will be sore, and there are likely to be times that you do not desire to complete your workout however, stick with the plan and you'll begin be amazed by the results you will see.

Chapter 5: Tips

In order to finish this book, I'd like to offer you some tricks and tips you can employ to aid you to succeed with my 21-day program that I've provided you with, by changing how you consume food and dropping those excess pounds.

One thing I'd like to address is the fact that you shouldn't alter the way you eat, but take to the challenge at while. Do you remember what I mentioned in the earlier chapters of my guide that once you cut out processed food items from your diet you'll be depressed? It is not a good idea to suffer from this when you attempt to tackle the task due to the fact that one of two modifications, if not both, is likely to fail.

It is better to alter the food you consume by removing processed foods out of your diet during the first 30 days. When you are able to get a grip of what you are putting into your body, you are able to focus on the 21-day program. There's no better option to drop the weight and maintain it off, than to do what you've learnt in this book. I would encourage you to test it out.

Another suggestion I'd like to share with you is to develop your own routine. You will need create a set daily time to perform every single cardio. Also, you must schedule an exact time every day for your intervals. If you say you'll do it sometime in the day, it won't take place. For you to make your own progress it is essential to create an action plan.

If you're just beginning to work out, divide your intervals over the course of your time of the day. If, for instance, an interval was five lunges, 5 pushups 5, 5 burpees and repeat five times, do it at different intervals throughout your entire day. This can help prevent your body to not feel overwhelmed. Also, it'll help you make sure that you don't get sore muscles early that could lead the person to quit.

If you find your muscles to be stiff, relaxing in a hot bath with a cup of Epsom salt can help ease muscles. It is also possible to eat more bananas, and protein powder to ease soreness in your muscles. Drinking water is among the most effective things that you can consume to keep muscle soreness at bay. This is something I can't emphasize enough. that you must ensure that you drink enough fluids.

You must ensure that you're having enough rest while you're going through this exercise. It is crucial to get enough sleep every day however, during massive lifestyle changes, you might discover that you require more rest. It is recommended to get 8-9 hours of rest per evening when going through the 21-day program so that you do not overwork your body.

You must be regular in your exercise schedule. If you only exercise once or twice a week, you will not be able get outcomes. If you wish to succeed with this challenge, it is important be consistent and complete all the tasks required during the exercise. When the challenge is finished, Do not think you have to quit your workout and get back to your normal way of life. It is your responsibility to decide to take the plunge and make changes to your lifestyle since if you go back to the old way of life, you'll only gain the weight that you have lost back, and shed the muscle you built up. It's not an easy task and, even while it's worthwhile to put effort into it the effort, it's not worthwhile if you decide to simply return to the previous routine.

Chapter 6: What is Calisthenics?

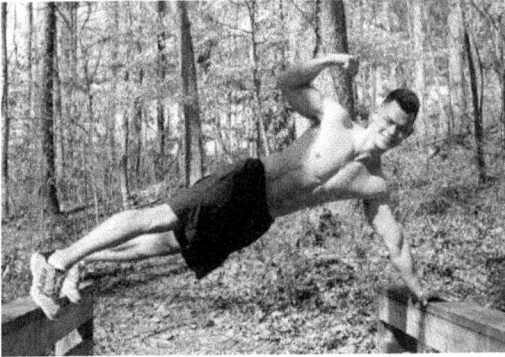

Calisthenics refers to a form of exercise which uses your body's weight in order to increase power. It increases your muscle mass and prepares your body for an athletic posture that is based on your personal characteristics and character. Calisthenics, a type of exercise which uses your body's weight and gravity in order to build muscles and boost fitness. It is derived out of the Greek words "Kalos" and "Stenos" The first meaning beauty and the other one meaning power (Thomas and. al., 2017). In addition to fitness, bodybuilding is commonly practiced by schoolchildren, for the gymnastics and outside practice.

One of the most well-known exercises in calisthenics includes Hannibal Lanham (Hannibal for King) He attracted the attention of millions of people to the discipline through his abilities in parks in Queens, New York.

Kenneth Gallarzo, the co-founder of the World Calisthenics Organization (WCO) began his career as an exercise instructor. He was intrigued by calisthenics following the sight of a fellow member at the gym performing an exercise that he'd previously never witnessed. When he began researching calisthenics Gallarzo discovered that the form of exercise provides a solid base for the other disciplines that build strength.

It's more than a commercial fitness program which promises much but does only a little. The research has proven that calisthenics increases body strength, composition and posture (Thomas and. al., 2017). The benefits that have been reported for calisthenics are many, and we will discuss them in greater detail when we get there.

The Benefits of Calisthenics

The body doesn't have to just move forward and backwards. Calisthenics includes twists, rotations pushing, pulling, leaps, squats, and other jumps to the movement. The exercises for Calisthenics will require more muscles to increase your muscle mass when you do them at a moderate or slow speed, and also more calories burning when performed at a slower pace and by doing more cardio. This is due to the fact that higher exercise intensity also boosts calories burned. The practice of calisthenics helps to build strength, become fitter and more slimmer. In addition the other benefits to these workouts:

* Flexibility. Since you don't require the equipment required for calisthenics it is possible to work out anywhere at any time. It is not necessary to stick to a specific schedule or set aside appointment to attend the gym. This is ideal if you're a busy person or have the same routine (although strongly recommended) can be a challenge for people

like you. You should instead make a place for freestyle fitness, which could include a frame that is functional and Swedish ladders. You can see that the only requirement with calisthenics is planning properly and perform the workouts in a disciplined manner the correct method.

A naturally toned body. The exercise will aid in burning fat, boost your strength and stamina, and build up the entire body. It can increase the production of endorphins. It will also help to feel more energetic. Calisthenics is a form of exercise that trains multiple muscles in the same session. In the case of push-ups, for example, they train the abdominal muscles, spine as well as the chest and arms. In this way you will appear more balanced and you'll never have to think about how to balance your workouts. The body will form and shape itself naturally, which is in line with your body shape, and your muscles will be at their best.

• Mindset changes. The exercise helps connect you to your body while increasing the physical awareness. Regular workouts may become monotonous and exercisers can lose their motivation. Calisthenics however, despite consisting of repetitions, can change the kinds of exercises and routines. When you have mastered one ability level, you can be able to move onto the next level. The challenges will increase as the body shape changes.

Then, last but certainly not the least, calisthenics can prevent injuries while exercising. The reason is that the exercises aren't designed to allow for over-training of a specific kind of muscle.

Calisthenics seem more appealing when you consider being able to avoid the expense of an gym membership, or exercise iron, or plan to your routine exercises. In the meantime performing exercises that mold your body naturally can be more healthy and offers greater mental and physical benefits over pumping iron.

What to do when you first start Calisthenics

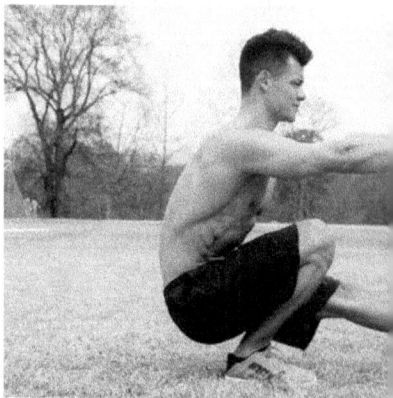

What should you do to start? This article will cover some of the fundamental principles of calisthenics, as well as the necessary elements you require to achieve a body transformation that is successful.

It's all about discovering the limits of your potential, expanding your boundaries and in a manner that is appropriate to your body's unique form and type. By achieving one goal following the next will provide you with a great strength and it will also become a great activity. Training with body weight is generally difficult to begin. Being unsure of things such as the best places to workout and the best way to start could be a challenge, however an appropriate mindset and understanding of exercises should assist begin.

If you choose to begin exercising with calisthenics you'll be in a dilemma about the best way to begin. Do you need to do some pushups and planks? Do you need to do more planning to your workouts to get the most effective results? A general rule is that most novices make mistakes that are easily corrected. The exercises are learned by repetition while the outcomes become apparent the more you work. In the beginning, you should focus on developing a positive mental attitude to learn and practice calisthenics.

Build Foundations: Earn Your Right to Progress

To earn your right to continue is first creating the basis for the long-term workout. Many people who are getting started with fitness become addicted to the first progress. The routines you're working on are improving each day. Your body and brain are receiving stimulation, and naturally, you want to push yourself further. But, it's essential to remain focused on your body, and to have the right direction in mind. Growing will begin to be demanding at one time or the next, and until you're prepared to face the obstacles, your motivation could fall.

How do you begin with calisthenics? While you may have come familiar with this notion from watching fitness professionals perform complex exercises, as a newbie will need to take it slow, in the interest for your health as well as security. It is recommended to start by doing basic exercises such as:

* Press-up. This workout can be modified for those who are new to the sport. If you want to do a beginner's push-up perform press-ups

by placing your hands placed on the bench with your feet on floor. When you've mastered this workout it is possible to progress to normal press-ups. Start by doing at least 20 reps.

* Dips. Once you've completed 20 press-ups you may start working on dips. For a dip, hold yourself onto a bar and then turn your elbows so that you dip, and then straighten them back upwards.

* Squats and lunges and planks.

* Rows. This is an workout where you are held onto an object, with the bar facing towards your chest and then do a backward lean, with your feet planted on the floor. Make sure you are as level to the ground as is possible.

Don't Compare Yourself to Others

The other rule is not to look at yourself in comparison to other people. The idea of comparing yourself with those who were earlier in their journey and have an extensive background using calisthenics may derail the motivation of your. Each person develops in their own way and on their own schedule. Additionally every body's constitution is unique. The age of your body, the health condition fitness history, your previous training experience, as well as the level of fitness you have will affect your stage of beginning as well as your exercise direction. Instead of comparing others' experiences with yours take inspiration from them and take their journey as a source of motivation to get to the direction you'd like to take.

Mix Strength with movement

Balance between fitness and mobility is essential ingredient to build the natural strength that lasts and energy. The majority of people concentrate on strength because it's the most sought-after objective to aim for. But, as you'll discover how to show your strength as well as what you're capable of doing by relying on the strength of your muscles. Balance and flexibility, coordination and the mental clarity you gain from exercises that are balanced will enhance your physical appearance as well as your overall performance. A balance of the strength and movement will allow you to be flexible and mobile throughout joints. In the beginning, if you're experiencing issues with your mobility, as typically happens to people who lead a more sedentary life, these exercises will assist you to increase your range of motion:

* Handstands. Handstands provide an exercise that improves the body's control and strength. In the absence of a solid experience in fitness handstands, you'll be able to master them once you've started of regular, beginner-level exercises. The risk of getting injured while doing handstands when you're an inexperienced person is minimal, as your hands will not have the strength to hold your body in a stable position unless the physical strength you have at present allows you to do it. There are a variety of variations to the exercise. Beginners should stick to the known as "line handstand", in where you hold your

body straight. The position can let your shoulders open, help improve your core strength and strengthen it and help ensure your back is protected. Over time, this practice helps you develop abilities that will be beneficial in various exercises.

Flags of humans. Are you thinking of turning your self into a flag? It's a good thing you'll enjoy trying it out, regardless of whether you don't succeed. Even though this may not be the easiest for beginners attempt, doing a basic variation is bound to keep your heart pumping it's an excellent practice. Prior to beginning practicing to fly the human flag, you should be able hold one arm for 30 seconds, perform the four sets of 10 pullups as well as hold a side-plank for 45 minutes. That's the core of the exercise, following which you'll practice by performing elbow side planks and sides planks that reach, inclined plansks on the sides (five sets that last 45 seconds on either side) and hanging hip hikers and shoulders push-ups pike (15-20 repetitions over a period of a minute).).

Trust Your Body

Since calisthenics workouts rely on only the strength and motion of the body. Your brain is able to keep you safe from injury through limiting moves that strain your body. The body won't utilize muscles that are rigid, or perform movements too difficult for your joints to avoid injuries and learning to pay attention to the body. The ability to move according to your physique and potential allows you to form a more appealing shape and utilize your power rather than limiting your movement.

The use of your body weight is one of the greatest benefits and the most challenging difficulties of calisthenics. It takes time to comprehend how your body adjusts and develops from producing resistance of its own. When you exercise, your body will become your own weight. As your body grows and gains in size, so does the amount of resistance. It is evident that it is an endless process that is abounds with possibilities for advancement.

The development of your calisthenics abilities will involve maintaining your joints. They'll be stretched more when you work out more vigorously. Flexibility and tension on your connective tissue will grow when you begin to develop your skills in calisthenics. As an example, if you perform pushups using the weight you started with then you'll have less weight, as opposed to a heavier body after some time of strengthening the muscles. This puts extra stress on joints, however they'll be slower to adjust to the change. The reason is that your muscles and ligaments don't receive the same blood flow that your muscles do.

Focus on Core Alignment

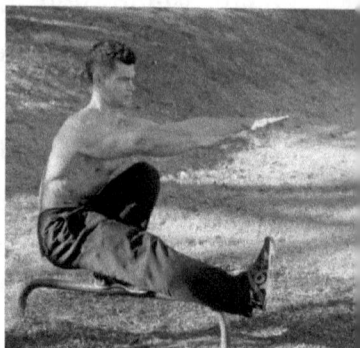

Traditional exercises employ various equipment and machines, however, calisthenics needs an alignment of your body in order to help support the weight of your body as well as to reap the greatest advantages. Aiming for body alignment is exercising your core every when you work out. For a proper use of your core adhere to the guidelines that are explained further in the book on how to ensure your body is aligned.

The shoulders of your body provide the most movement range, and they allow for a variety of motions. Yet, their stability requires enhancement through a regular workout. Shoulder exercises are among your top priorities. Setting and pushing your shoulders, along with pulling are crucial. The practice of opposing motions can help keep your movement stable.

Hands that are balanced is an crucial component of fitness. To do this, try frog stand exercises in the beginning. Then, progress to handstands, tiger bends as well as elbow levers and others that are more difficult exercises.

When you're done with the day, the journey you've taken ought to be exciting and uplifting. If you are bored, it is an indication to change your routine and add different, challenging workouts. Now you know what calisthenics actually is, and the things you must accomplish before starting exercising. However, wait! There's still time to get started with any workouts. There's plenty to master for the best, well-planned fitness regimen and diet plan that yields healthy, noticeable effects. In the next chapter, we will shed some more information on the calisthenics rules to be followed for a safe and safe exercises.

Chapter 7: Calisthenics Principles

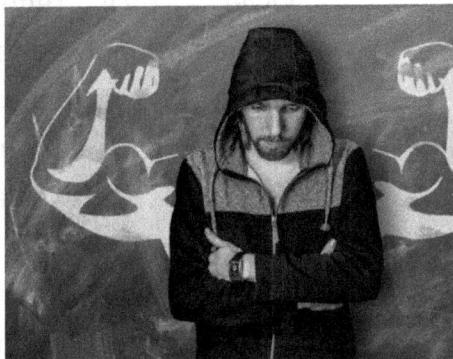

Once you have a basic understanding of the calisthenics concept and its benefits over weightlifting and weight lifting, let us discuss the calisthenics concepts in depth. The principles of calisthenics will show you how to organize your exercises and workouts in order to achieve the most effective results, as well as how to conquer some of the obstacles associated with this notion. There are many exercise plans available, all created to provide the best outcomes for various kinds of people and groups. For any exercise program to be effective, it should recognize the distinct particulars of every person. The exercise plan you choose to follow will be based on your personal needs and physique. In the case of example, if you're trying to improve your power, you'll require distinct exercise regimen as opposed to if you wanted to build muscle. This is dependent on your overall health as well as your previous experiences with exercise, as well as how long you're able to spend on exercise. The following general guidelines when you exercise can help you create an effective workout program and get better results.

Once you start calisthenics your entire lifestyle will change. Like any other change it is important to establish upon solid foundations to ensure long-term success and sustainable for the long haul. The practice of calisthenics goes beyond just exercise It's a lifestyle.

In this article in this chapter, we'll go over the fundamental principles or the underlying concepts of calisthenics. We will discuss the terms that are most commonly used and the specific issues that every person who performs calisthenics is faced with and the best way to solve the issue. The course will cover the fundamental rules and aspects that beginners must learn and be aware of. Three fundamental rules of exercising that are applicable to everyone regardless of levels, comprise:

Overload

The principle of adaptation happens when your body is under more tension or pressure than is normal. If you put your body under stress by putting it through a higher level of performance and greater stress on the body, it'll enhance its capabilities to meet these requirements. This is why overload is a stimulant that is essential for results during exercise. In the absence of it, you'll only notice slight to moderate improvement. The body adapts to the strains it is put under to be able to deal with it better each moment, which makes your muscles grow as they get bigger. This is evident at a cellular level by enhancing the cardiovascular efficiency of people who train frequently and intensively. That's how your physical fitness levels rise, resulting through faster and improved fitness levels, as well as bigger more powerful, more defined muscles. This article will show you how to modify overload and achieve the desired outcomes.

Do you workout regularly? Regularity introduces consistency to your workout routine. The general rule is that exercises are followed by time for recuperation. This balances out the strain and permits the body to recover from the strain and to adjust to changing conditions that are essential in order to achieve some results. The training phase are best followed by a period that allow you to notice results. both are vital. Training and recovery both require proper nutrition as well as quality sleep. A healthy diet provides sufficient energy for exercising and recovery, a good night's sleep can help your body to heal and recuperate.

The level of intensity you exercise in is also crucial. There must be a equilibrium in intensity workout to create enough tension to achieve the desired results, however not enough to cause injury or burnout. The principle is that intensity is increased by either raising resistance or the repetitions. Be aware that too many repetitions can interfere with increasing strength. It is better to incorporate exercises, switch exercises, or alter your tempo in order to boost intensities of training.

Exercise duration depends on exercise intensity. It is recommended that more vigorous workouts to be done in shorter durations while less intense exercises that last longer. You will get enough energy without overdosing.

SAID Principle

The SAID principle refers to Specific adaptation to the demands of society. This is a principle that requires focusing on certain goals or actions that help improve the abilities. This is a principle that states that the kind of change that occurs from exercise is dependent on the level of strain placed on a specific part of the body. It could be a muscles, or a group. In order to achieve your objectives through exercising, you'll select which exercises to execute based on the results you're aiming for. An example of distinct outcomes could be wanting to be an elite runner or trying to shed weight and increase your the health of your. The first one is ideal if you do outdoor sprinting and running, while the latter requires a greater focus on cardiovascular fitness, muscle strength as well as lifestyle adjustments. The way to put it, your workout sessions must be in line to your desired goals.

SAID is also a sign that your body is equipped with the capacity to change to biomechanical and neurological demands that are placed on it. This means that you must do your best instead of working hard and blindly. The SAID principle should be the basis for your decision-making.

Note: You should not pick your activities randomly. Select activities based on science that are proven to be effective.

* Adjustment to: Be sure of what type of adaptation you would like to see happen in this portion of your learning.

* Implied: The activities have to be conducted consistently for the specified time period.

*Requirements: Do the activity(s) at a sufficient level of intensity that you can achieve the change you want, and while doing the task safely and correctly.

Progressive Overload

The idea of progressive overload implies that you gradually intensify the pressures you place on your muscle and skeletal system. By doing this, you can improve endurance, strength as well as muscle mass. In order to build strength and strengthen your muscles, it is necessary to continue to make your muscles perform harder than previously. Once you get your muscles comfortable, for instance lifting a certain weight or performing an workout, you'll add weight or intensify repetitions or sets in order in order to force your muscles to perform harder.

The exercise you do will need gradually become more challenging in order to reach higher levels of performance. In the event that you do not intensify your exercise slowly, you'll hit a plateau. For good results, you must go through a process of load, while an extensive alteration will require a lot of focused effort. The most basic exercises for resistance are broken down into:

* Multi-joint workouts, which are also called core exercises including squats. They require you to stabilize your back to maintain your spine in a neutral posture. These are often referred to as exercises for structural stability. Squats, for instance is a strain on the spine and demands the core muscles in order to keep it in place. Additionally, it engages the hip, ankle and knee joints, and places an additional strain on gluteus maximus and

quadriceps muscles, and the hamstring muscles.

* Core exercises may be further broken down using an increase in the speed of movement. These are the so-called explosive or power, exercises are carried out at greater speeds.

Exercises for single joints, or assist exercises. The exercises only target one joint, and they recruit one or more small or larger muscles.

Leverage Training: Body Vs. Machines

Utilizing your body weight for workout, rather than machines it is a feasible and natural method to exercise. The practice of using your body to leverage is becoming very popular due to it being extremely effective, as well as because it can be done whenever, wherever as a solo or in the company of others.

Reps and Sets

Here are the numbers of sets and reps you should perform in your leverage training, to meet the goals you have set for yourself.

* Strength 5 reps

* Power 2 to 4 repetitions

* Endurance: 15 reps

* Hypertrophy 8-12 reps

Resistance

The term "resistance" refers to the fact that you employ an external type of resistance in order to tighten the muscles in order to increase tone as well as strengthening, building up muscles, and for endurance training. It's great that you don't require gymnasium equipment to do the same results with calisthenics. It is possible to use your personal body weights or a collection of resistance band, or perhaps grab a couple cans of food off the shelf of the pantry. In essence, whatever is useful to cause your muscles work will help.

Some examples of good calisthenics resistance training equipment are:

* Bands of resistance. They provide excellent resistance when stretched like around legs or arms.

* Any type of suspension device. Rings and suspension bars as well as a solid tree branch can be used. Your own physique weight as well as gravity to complete the workouts.

* Free weights using the standard equipment used for strengthening consisting of dumbbells, kettlebells as well as barbells. A few sandbags can work similarly.

* The use of medicine balls is in a great way for resistance training. They are suitable to all stages of fitness and ages.

* Weight only. Building the perfect physique need not need a gym and all the equipment stacked up there. The only thing that is required is your strength and endurance. It is possible to perform chin-ups push-ups and squats wherever or at any time. You do not require a fitness membership to perform this. Resistance training using body weight is great

on trips, be it to work or just for pleasure You don't have to haul bags filled with heavy equipment with you.

Top Three Problems and How to Resolve Them

Beginners face three challenges as drawbacks or obstacles, once beginning their calisthenics training. However, it's not all that bad because the solution is to accept the issue to heart, find solutions and then implement them.

Freedom

Sure, it may sound weird, but the independence of calisthenics has its own drawbacks. It is not necessary to a exercise facility and you are able to do the workout wherever you want. Also, you are not governed to a schedule or time limit and aren't committing the time to use machines. Some people find this may not be a good thing as they have trouble sticking to a regimen. It could result in inconsistentness with their exercise routines. On the other hand, the opposite aspect is a possible scenario because you are able to workout virtually anyplace and at any time, which means you could fall victim to the trap of exercising excessively, often.

Variety

The old saying, that variation is the spice in life is absolutely true. As an example there are 21 methods of doing push-ups but if you're aware of the three or two ways you can complete them, then your workout routines can become monotonous. It's important to incorporate diversification into your training because the moment boredom starts to creep in, it may result in depression.

This is another reason why you may be on the opposite side of the spectrum, and you'd like to attempt all possible variations of every exercise. It means that you're not focused on a single kind of workout, however, you are working out in a random manner. This can negatively affect the way you would like for your progress to follow. It can certainly be difficult for newbies however, as with all things in life, it is important to discover a way to remain motivated and stay on your path that you've chosen.

Simplicity

The simplicity of calisthenics could cause problems for certain individuals. Some people find it hard to overcome plateaus that can last several months and they get bored of following a pre-determined exercise routine. Many feel that unless they utilize equipment and tools and equipment, they're not making notable gains. If you feel you're getting bored, then it's an ideal time to alter some aspects to your fitness routine.

The Solutions to These Problems

For you to resolve these issues You must create an organized and disciplined exercise plan that keeps you in the right direction and never stop moving.

Make a routine for your workouts from the point you're at, and focus on the direction you'd like to go.

Create a strategy in pencil or on your laptop, then make it available for printing. It's important to keep an image of your objectives and the exercises that are going to help you reach your targets.

Be sure to include your exercise routine within your schedule for each day when it is convenient that works for you.

This will help you sharpen your attention and prevent the temptation to do over or under.

Key Rules and Focal Points

In this entire volume, we'll repeat the fact that calisthenics is much more than just a physical workout. It's a brain and body experience. When you are able to master your body, the mind is playing a significant role in the process so you are able to enjoy all the advantages of calisthenics. Therefore, it is crucial to get your body and mind in the right balance before you begin in calisthenics.

Patience and Consistency

A majority of people lack an excessive amount of patience for everything they undertake. They're eager to get things done and be able to see results immediately. Two things that beginners must remember in all instances is patience and consistent. If you do not cultivate patience through your training and putting in the effort to achieve your goals. You will experience a lack of consistency in your workouts as you seek immediate results and you begin to feel depressed. It's all about persistence and perseverance.

No Cheating

There aren't any quick fixes or shortcuts to follow when it comes to the exercises. Your body is a magnificent biomechanical machine that is designed to perform an incredible variety of types of motion. For you to achieve your goals, and reap the long-lasting benefits of calisthenics you have be focused on achieving all the motions that the body has to offer. Doing a sloppy job and taking shortcuts will not work and you're only making yourself look bad. Concentrate on each workout in a perfect way, and try to be sure to do it every when you exercise. Don't cheat yourself. It is worth all of your effort at every opportunity.

Set Realistic Goals

If you begin using calisthenics brand new and you can see improvement with each workout. This can be a really exciting moment, and you've got every right to be enjoying the moment. As time passes, however the body gets more fit and strong the rate at which you improve is likely to slow. It's normal, but for you to stay away from disappointment, it is important establish realistic expectations of your goals within a realistic workout schedule.

Stop Comparing Yourself to Others

In the beginning as a beginner, you'll be performing generalized exercises. It's the way it should be. Through generalization, it is possible to get to know and decide if you're looking towards becoming a specialist. You could, for instance, choose a specific area of interest and become specialized in handstands. You shouldn't be comparing yourself to any other person, particularly not one who's been practicing calisthenics over a period of time and has a specialization in the field, as you place too much stress on you. Being a generalist means you'll perform a variety of workouts whereas the specialist will focus on a specific area. You'll be slow to progress due to the fact that your focus is more broad, which is perfectly normal and not something to be concerned about.

Utilize social media in a rational way to gain more information and suggestions. Avoid comparing yourself to celebrities who post and brag about their achievements and successes. While you can appreciate that people like them work tirelessly to accomplish their personal targets, since that's real, but don't consider them as a benchmark to measure your performance. Social media can do less harm to novices, as well as to experienced people who practice calisthenics. Celebrity hype in general could undermine confidence in oneself. The goal of calisthenics is to become the most effective you can be, and not become like any other person.

Maintain Diet and Lean Muscle Weight

Diet plays an enormous part in the progress you make in calisthenics. There is no way to increase your calisthenics performance by having junk food in your diet, or by eating huge quantities of food. This is simply not possible like this. It is essential to maintain and attain the weight of lean muscles by following a proper training regimen as well as a healthy diet. The weight of your body is not able to replace the lean muscle mass. The food you eat and the exercise program should be in alignment with the objectives you wish to attain.

Proper Training Plan

There must be a carefully designed training plan that is worked to meet your requirements and objectives. It is not enough to just fumble around performing random exercises hoping to reap any benefit. If you don't have a plan for training You will be enticed by the trap of simply following what you feel is the most easy to accomplish and then what pops into your head. It is then up to you to do whatever you like to do during your workout routine and not think about the things you must complete to meet your objectives. The practice of grabbing random workouts for training can lead to an unplanned progression that leads the user nowhere.

Develop a program of training that you stick to for at least 6 weeks prior to reassessing your objectives. It is then your decision whether you would like to stick on this specific program of training and then move onto an alternative.

Stomp Your Ego Down

Ego is not a valid factor in any type of training for physical fitness It is definitely in the case with calisthenics. It is the same for both men and women. It is not a good idea to allow your self-esteem to take over your life. What you'll end up doing is a sprain or injury. It will put your training back and make it challenging to reach the goals you set. Take a lesson from those who've let their egos cut off their reasoning. You can stomp your ego to the ground and perform calisthenics in the correct way with a minimum of overextending your limits.

Chapter 8: Flexibility and Mobility

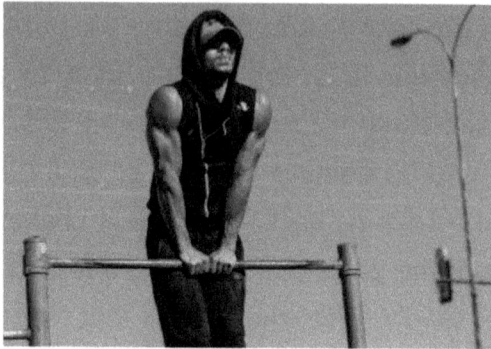

The flexibility and mobility of joints are usually neglected in the fitness world. The diet, strength of muscles and the definition of muscle strength, loss in weight as well as other aspects of training are often more important than taking note of the flexibility of joints and muscles. But, mobility and flexibility are more important than many people are aware. They ease pain from daily exercises, and are crucial in maintaining heart health. Many people are suffering of low back pain that is chronic, that is the result of inflexibility and lack of mobility within the body and tight hamstrings.

An unhealthy lifestyle leads the lower back area to become round, which impacts tension from body weight in the lower back. This creates discomfort. Inability to move your lower back can lead to lower productivity and decreased productivity at work as well.

The study also showed that flexibility can be linked with death. The more inflexible people are, the greater the risk of developing cardiovascular diseases. Mobility and flexibility both relate to joints to be able to move an array of movements. It can also decrease because of muscle tightness that prevent proper exercise and can increase the likelihood for injury. Research has also shown that exercises for flexibility and mobility are precautionary measures against injuries but not just when an injury happens.

Flexibility and Mobility Exercises

Moving your body will assist in preventing Injuries as well as increasing your strength. If you're a novice in calisthenics you're likely interested in the variety of exercises that you could complete and the number of repetitions that produce the desired results. This is completely normal, however longer-term balance and strength will require you to exercise flexibility and mobility. Mobility is comprised of two distinct elements of flexibility:

Flexibility that is passive: Low stress muscles, tendon and ligament flexibility. This is similar to running splits while on the ground.

* Dynamic Flexibility: High-stress flexible ligaments, tendons and muscles. Engaging in dynamic flexibility exercises is essential for improving fitness levels and ensure flexibility when under tension. It requires a lot of endurance in addition to exercising muscles and ligaments. In essence, your muscles should not be your sole point to focus on when you exercise. Your ligaments and tendons need equal care, because they're subjected to equally under stress during exercise, however they require more time to heal and adjust.

Whatever your strength in muscles it is possible to get hurt when you perform everyday activities when your ligaments aren't flexible enough. The problem of poor mobility can be fixed by a variety of stretching exercises that are designed to enhance the flexibility of your. Even though they can seem dull as they aren't designed to build muscle strength or build muscles but they're essential to be healthy in the long term. Utilizing your bodyweight can help with to achieve this because your body is able to maintain balance and, like I mentioned previously, will not allow you to perform movements which could cause injury to the body. What can you accomplish to enhance flexibility? There are several kinds of exercises you could perform:

* Active stretching. Extensive exercises for the shoulders comprise back levers and V sits and skinning cats. These exercises stretch muscles tight that are in your hands and shoulders especially on your biceps. These muscles can hinder stretching your shoulders correctly. These muscles will allow you to extend your

arms on the back of your arms as well as aid exercises that use weights.

* Active shoulder stretching. Engaging in exercises that cause tight shoulders are not just a way to decrease their effectiveness, but could may also result in tearing muscles and rupture of muscles and tendons. For example, exercises like V-sits and German hangs, especially those with more sophisticated versions, require lots of flexibility in the shoulders.

What do your stretches should be in the form of a picture? Begin slowly by doing three sets of one-minute hold every week, 3 times. Once you've gained movement and experience then you can concentrate on the more German hangings (skinning cats) and begin with three to five half-minute hold. After you've learned the basics of stretching, it's time to proceed to challenging warm-up exercises for example:

* Motion range exercises. The exercises involve joints in the full range of motions.

There is no need for tension to be extreme when doing these exercises but they're nevertheless important. They include exercises for mobility that target shoulders, like the ones listed below.

The shoulder is dislocated. The exercises are easy that can significantly increase the flexibility of your shoulders. For these exercises require a broad grip on a lightweight bar or dowel rod. While your arms are raised to your sides and elbows extended, you can move the rod as far and over your head as you can. The bar should be between five and ten pounds. If it is lighter, the workout turns into the passive flexibility. This is where you need to stretch muscles too in addition to ligaments and joints. For beginners begin using a larger grip, and move your hands closer when you advance. If you can complete this exercise using hands that are a little distance from your shoulders and elbows, raise the weight of the rod, and then return to using the wider grip. The flexibility will improve when you push yourself to the limit but progress can only be accomplished by increasing the weight, and then starting again.

The primary goal of this workout is to help you to attain a full shoulder blade or the scapula's movement. The scapula must protract while your arms outwards and your shoulders should extend. After that, they will recline when you lift your arms and push the shoulders back towards your head. Dislocated shoulders aren't speed training they should be performed gradually and with patience.

* Eating the cats. It's not literal, but it's a good idea. This workout mimics the body position of the animal that is in this scenario, and is easier and less demanding than it seems. The method involves hanging from an exercise bar that pulls you up and lifting your body upwards and then directly in front of the person. Practice the move as far as you can before slowly getting back to the starting posture. In the beginning, it may be slow and challenging when you're just beginning however that's not an issue. This workout

requires lots of strength as well as flexibility so you must take your time before you're ready to do the an Instagram-worthy number of repetitions. You'll improve your ability after you've repeated the workout. In order to practice in a safe manner the shoulder blades must be in a slight retraction when being suspended from a bar as well as before beginning the move. By doing this, you'll be able to raise your body with ease before you begin the exercise.

Distractions to your shoulders. This workout doesn't help bring your shoulders within their complete movement range. The exercise stretches ligaments as it takes away your upper arm bone away from the joint capsule. The workout is pleasant, regardless of the possibility of injury. For this the right way, use an amount of 5-10 pounds, and then be able to bend. The non-swinging arm should be placed on a stool, after that, relax and then swing the other hand by circling it either counter-clockwise or clockwise. While doing this exercise synovial fluid is lubricates the joint, making it more elastic. It should, however, be performed slowly and with patience. Avoid rushing or using a full range. The goal of this exercise is to distract your muscles of the humerus, and increase flexibility on your shoulders. It's impossible to overdo the exercise. Ideally, you'll be doing the exercise every day and for as long as you want.

Moving exercises can be a good warming up before handstands and they should be performed with two-minute intervals.

A lack of flexibility may not only hinder your mobility however, it can also cause you to feel slow and stiff. Whatever your strength level the lack of flexibility could hinder your fitness and everyday routine activities. After you've established a solid base with pull-ups, push-ups and dips, further advancement will require greater agility and flexibility. More difficult exercises like those with the lever back, muscle-up and L-sits require you to add the flexibility routine to your routine. The stretching exercises you do will allow you to perform more complex moves such as:

* Better Front Fold exercises. This helps assist in making handstands, hang leg lifts Vsits and L-sits more comfortable. The exercises may look as though they just work the core muscles, however that's far from the truth. They require also the posterior chain to move. The foot folds let you combat gravity, without adding additional muscle tension. The tightness of the hamstrings and feet is usually seen in novices while straightening your legs when doing an L-sit seems impossible regardless of your strength. Strength alone will not guarantee an appropriate V- or L-sit with out flexibility training. If you are able to focus on strengthening your hamstrings as well as the flexibleness of your back fold and back fold, resistance wlthin these regions will be reduced. In order to do these exercises properly start by straightening your legs while in a pike posture on the ground. To begin, perform them while keeping your back in a round position in the beginning, then flatten

your back when you move on to the next exercises. The exercises might need a lengthy warm-up.

Overhead Mobility

The exercises for overhead mobility loosen those muscles at the rear of your arms as well as your upper back as well as your shoulders. Active stretching exercises can increase your mobility overhead and will aid in the upper body, such as handstands. To do this, try these two exercises

* Chin-up dead hang which can stretch your shoulders through external rotation. The basic dead hang offers multiple benefits, ranging from releasing the spine and stretching the muscles in the back, arm, as well as the core muscle. For a dead hang take a seat on a bench. Then, hold a safe overhead bar by using both your hands. The hands must be shoulder width to each other. Get off the bench and grasp the bar. Maintain a comfortable position for 10 seconds, and then for up to one minute as long as you can. Go

back to your bench and repeat the exercise up to 3 times. If you're not sure if your body shape can quite yet allow this type of exercise You can remain on the bench and move by grasping the bar and lift your chin to the ceiling. It is then possible to hang on the bar, with your feet sitting upon the bench.

* Hanging cobra where you'll need rings for gymnastics. Adjust the rings' size in line with your chest. Grab the rings using your hands. As you sink into your hand position, do it slowly, first sliding on your knees and after that, pulling your legs and feet backwards to the extended position. Next, you can twist slightly, initially to the side that is stiffer first, then the opposite side. You should hold the position the longest time you are able to and as long as you feel comfortable. It is also possible to lift your shoulders upwards and hold it for three to five seconds and afterwards, ease into the position. Do this for three to five times, and then switch onto the next position then repeat. When you are done, go back to the hang position, keeping

your hands in alignment with your shoulders, with your head positioned parallel to your hands. Do this for several seconds before getting away from the posture. This is a great exercise for people suffering from back or lower-back pain or anybody who would like to stretch the upper back, hands as well as their chest and lower abdominal.

Calisthenics exercises that involve head-to-head movements, for example, handstands need a lot of shoulder flexibility. Like you've learned before, muscles that are stiff can hinder the range of motion, but they also can increase your risk of getting injured. In addition, it ensures the stability of your shoulders during exercise and flexing your overhead properly as well as the capacity to stretch your elbows, while ensuring the strength of your spine and core. You can see that the body and all of its parts have a connection, and one cannot function without the flexibility and strength of the next.

The upper body workouts can work the shoulder blade, as well regardless of whether exercises focus on your shoulders directly. Due to this, your ability to hold your posture in a stable manner is dependent on the stability of your shoulders and flexibility. Shoulder stability is crucial as well as range of motion in order in order to prevent a slumped or sagging body. Three more simple exercises that you can do to increase your range of motion overhead:

• Shoulder mobilization. This exercise is simple: make a circle around your shoulder throughout the entire movement. Do you feel tension or crackling? You can then circle until your capula turns smoothly and easily!

* Active range of motion. Now, you should rotate your shoulder by fully extending the arm and use your entire range of movement. This will improve the body's alignment while doing handstands.

* Shoulder extension using the help of a band. This exercise is for beginners. It's simple and

enjoyable, and you'll be a great workout even if you suffer as a result of spending for hours in front of a computer. Stand on a band and hold the upper portion of the band using your hands. Spread the band across your head with your fingers aligned with shoulders. After that, extend your shoulders as high as you are able, and then lower them, and return them up until the shoulders remain in a relaxed position. This workout also works the lower abdominal as well as your lower back muscles. by gently stretching the muscles in your arms. If you are sitting on your feet you can also stretch your the lower back muscles as well as joints.

Chapter 9: Safety, Rest, and Recovery

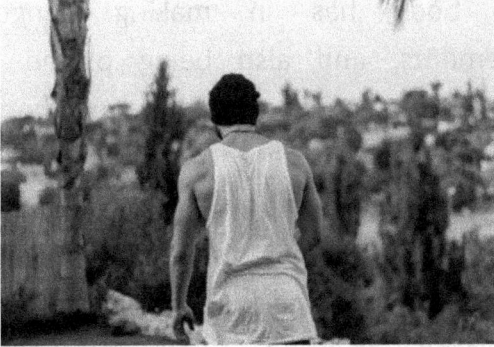

In the preceding section, you were taught about the importance of flexibility as well as mobility to reduce the risk of injury. While stretching does not guarantee the best results or security from injuries. Recovery and rest are important for the most physical and mental health benefits. In this section we'll explain how the benefits of rest and recovery are greater fitness outcomes, as well as the best ways to take a break in order to let your muscles get stronger and bigger.

Safety: How to Prevent Injury in Calisthenics

The prevention of injuries is a vital element of every exercise. Although calisthenics is not a risk of injury because of the limitations that your body has in making dangerous movements, and also being placed in a position that is unhealthy however, there are some ways to take care to reap the maximum gains from exercising and avoid overtraining. The practice of using your body weight can help prevent overuse as compared to risk associated with lifting weights.

The calisthenics program puts less strain on joints, and could cause less injury However, injuries can be a possibility if you're not vigilant enough. Knowing how to avoid injury during calisthenics training is crucial in order to make progress in a steady manner. For your convenience, there are only two basic preventive strategies you could employ when doing calisthenics. This is what you should take to avoid straining yourself too much while exercising:

* Warm-up. Don't begin a workout by not warming up for at minimum 10 minutes. The practice of using bodyweights is believed as light enough to not needing warm-ups for novices, so taking an extra 10 minutes for it might seem like removing time of your workout routine. However, this isn't the case. Properly warming up will help the speed of your workout and make it simpler and more fun. I provided a couple of exciting warm-ups for mobility and flexibility in my previous section. You can, however, pick any warm-up routine that you enjoy. The process of warming up will allow blood flow to begin flowing through joints, lubricating joints to avoid the risk of injury.

Try to practice with a ball. Calisthenics does not require a lot of equipment or aids for lifting, however, a few useful instruments, including a lacrosse ball is one of them. helps you get the most exercise as well as performance. The use of a lacrosse ball can be beneficial for protecting joints from injuries, especially the ones in your elbows as well as wrists. Massage these regions by using a ball made of lacrosse helps alleviate joint pain as well as ease the strain on these regions. It is easy to relieve the muscle or joint discomfort by pressing the ball in those areas where you feel tension, soreness or tension. If you practice this routinely it will help you avoid the joint and muscle soreness that occurs after a workout.

Make use of variations. Begin with less challenging variations of the more challenging exercises in order to give your joints and muscles time to get warm. As an example, if you plan to perform handstands, try a few of standard push-ups before you begin. A couple of times suffice to adapt your body's response to the motion. So, you can be able to avoid straining joints too much.

* Move the target area around. It is important to switch your exercises so that you concentrate on various muscle groups during the workout. By doing this, muscles are prevented from becoming accustomed to a

particular exercise, which can reduce the efficiency of that movement. In addition, you'll be able to be able to avoid putting too much strain on joints. This could occur if you perform repeatedly the same workout. To avoid this, you need to think of two different exercises per week. Make plans for two distinct exercises that target the specific muscle groups as well as rotating these exercises. It will prevent your from becoming bored by the exercises. This can be the case if you do the same workout routine session after session, and week following week.

Concentrate on your specific skills. Calisthenics differs from weight training in numerous aspects, with one being that it progresses because of improved physical abilities rather than a rush to complete the number of repetitions and exercises. The focus on learning the physical aspects of your movements instead of focusing on external outcomes, changes your attention on the physical look of your body the feeling of an natural desire to increase your body's structure and movement. In this way, when you examine your arm like, for instance, you don't focus on what you would like your biceps or triceps muscles to appear like. If you are focused on increasing the weight of your exercises as well as increasing repetitions, it is difficult to consider how this aligns with your specific body and overall health. The result could be injury.

Instead, think about what kind of move you're attempting to master as well as ways to improve how to master it. Muscles will improve by this method most likely However, focussing on precision of movements as well as the correct posture and the alignment of your body can provide greater physical outcomes as well as greater advantages for your health. This also helps prevent injuries since your thoughts are centered around your body's needs and the limits for your own body.

Calisthenics Rest and Recovery

If you're looking to strengthen your muscles to become more flexible and healthy as well as improve your overall appearance and well-being, then stopping could be a bit odd. It's difficult to resist the urge to train if you're bursting with motivation, enjoy exercising, and are getting the first signs of results. Rest and recuperation are essential. They enable the connective tissue and muscles to grow and recover in addition to avoiding the risk of overload. Let us take a look at how.

If you do your exercise properly as well as with the most efficient exercise regimen the muscles and connective tissues are subject to micro-tears. These minor injuries to muscles can cause an increase in muscle mass, as your human body "fills" these tears to repair the muscle and cause it to increase in the size. But, it's not possible to do this or at the very least, not in a healthy way in the absence of rest and recuperation. It's as simple as that Put stress and strain onto your muscles and create tiny tears. after that, rest and let them heal, and your muscles develop.

The premise behind rest and recuperation is easy to grasp, however its implementation generally isn't. Exercisers who are new to calisthenics tend to be puzzled about when and for how long they need to exercise and when to recover and rest afterwards. Another issue that confuses exercisers include the right diet for rest and workout days that we'll tackle within the subsequent chapters.

At this point we should focus on the necessity of recovery and rest. Although you may feel wonderful after a long and intense exercise, however your body is really, exhausted and depleted. This happens following exercise the body and your brain start to adjust to new conditions. When the brain is aware of intense physical strain, it'll start a process of adaptation when you're on rest. If you fail to get enough rest, you're at risk of injuries. If you train consistently during long durations and you're at risk of injuring your body to the point that you're in a position to not train for a period of up to one year.

Calisthenics can put an enormous amount of strain on the body. This adds strain not just to your muscles as well as connective tissue as well as wrists and ligaments. You've already heard that it takes them nearly two times longer to heal as in comparison to muscles. People who exercise regularly often have elbow pain or arm pain. In the event of this one way to alleviate discomfort is to take a break from exercising for a few minutes and then rest. It will ease the tension caused by injured tissues. If you are able to rest frequently after exercising for a period of weeks or months and years, you'll be able work out for a long time without suffering injury. If you do suffer serious injuries, they might hinder you from doing exercise all over.

There are a variety of reasons people aren't able to relax. For some, they fear being unable to train will cause their muscles weaker, or cause them to put pounds to gain it back. Some people simply want to grab every opportunity to grow or improve their skills, or developed a habit of training as it's enjoyable and rewarding. If you're preparing for the event of your choice, it's not impossible that a deadline could push the limits of your training.

All of these arguments tend to be hard to resist but there are a variety of legitimate reasons to take an absence, even if you are uneasy about it. To begin, taking for up to a week's relaxation won't cause you decrease your strength. In fact, you may get stronger due to the process of adaptation. If you take a break the muscles recover and expand. But, you must modify your diet according to changing conditions to prevent excess weight increase.

A structured rest schedule can assist you in getting more outcomes. When you are resting often and frequently between exercise Your muscular and neuromuscular system will be better able to adapt to the stress that is being put on them. The process is known as supercompensation. It's a biological response that takes place in the event that you are greater in strength than before.

If you get dependent on exercise, it may turn into a risky and harmful habit both mentally and physically. A break from exercising will allow the body and mind to get a more complete awareness and stability.

If you're in the process of preparing to participate in a sporting event or contest the exercise routine you're following must include adequate time for rest. If you do not get enough rest, it could affect the quality of your work. Once you understand the reasons why you need to rest and recover, let's talk about what you need to do to relax and recover after training correctly.

How to Plan Calisthenics Rest Days

It is important to plan your relaxation days in accordance with the goals of your workout and their level of intensity. The more frequent and rigorous your exercise routine, the greater time you will need for rest and adaptation. Therefore, the days off for rest should be equally divided throughout the week's schedule.

What are Rest Days?

Like the title suggests that rest days are weeks when there is no exercising. It is important to be reasonable and flexible in planning your days off. This is a very personal issue, so you must make time to consider which days you will rest. second or even every other day. It will be contingent on your activities and lifestyle as well as your ability to recover in general, as well as your work schedule. But, the plan should not be too rigid. It is important to allow yourself time to relax if you find yourself in need of to do so.

What are the steps to take when with your ideal plan for rest? Standard exercise programs that are designed for exercisers who regularly do their routines might not work for those who are new to calisthenics. Therefore, you'll require a slower speed. When you're only beginning with your ligaments, muscles and tendons may need to rest longer in comparison to experienced athletes. In order to avoid injury It's a good idea to choose longer periods of rest between exercises for the upper body.

Apart from that the other thing to consider is planning for de-loading weeks. This plan should be executed over four weeks, which means that week 4 is lighter and less intense in comparison to the three previous weeks. However, this doesn't suggest that your workouts should be overly light or you have to not train at all during that week. Training intensity will be sufficient to sustain your progress, but at less exercise and the stress. In this week, you should concentrate more on stretching and mobility. Be assured that these low-stress workouts will not harm your overall performance. It's likely that once having followed the right program, you'll be healthier and more flexible.

The chapter in this section, you've learned more about the importance of recovery and rest when it comes to calisthenics. When you take a break the body can be able to recover and improve itself. It's not the time you don't have for exercising. As we've all learned, if work out continuously and do not take breaks this can weaken the body, and eventually cause muscle injury. The resting days you learned about are essential for physical and mental motives. Not only do your muscles require the time to recover and build however, you need some time to let loose from the stress of working out, as well as to manage training with work and home. If you aren't getting enough rest it is possible to be suffering from the syndrome of overtraining.

In the course of your study, recovery is where your body adjusts to stress this is the moment that muscle strength and growth occur. Also, this is the best moment to replenish the sweat-loss water to prevent dehydration and to allow muscle cells to replenish glycogen stores and energy reserves and to grow through the repair of tissues that have been damaged. Short-term, recovery is a good way to give you energy for longer-term training and improve your performance. Over time, it'll aid your body in adapting to exercise, and aid to strengthening your muscles, so that you are able to progress.

Chapter 10: Rebalance the Scales

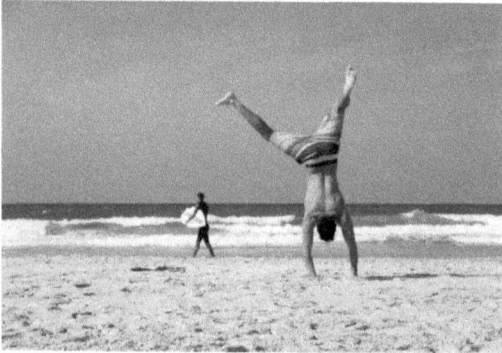

Calisthenics is an training that incorporates the power of endurance, strength, mobility as well as gymnastic exercises all under the same umbrella. In our introduction we talked about the reasons this kind of exercise is a favorite among so numerous people with different types of fitness, ages, and health status.

The thing that makes calisthenics unique is that it's not just exercise that offers an array of benefits to every participant It is an entire lifestyle shift. When their bodies undergo physical changes the way they eat is altered, and they lead an improved and more active life. Their emotional and mental wellbeing improve in the same way, and they manage everything they do with a sense of mindfulness.

Life Lessons

The word calisthenics refers to an amalgamation of Greek words that mean beauty and strength. The term strength refers at physical strength and beauty is the appealing external appearance of someone. However however, these terms refer to many more things than mere physical characteristics. Consider the power of determination even in the face of hardship as well as the pleasure of giving someone a hug without seeking anything back.

Physical calisthenics helps practitioners learn basic life skills, which don't require physical strength or strength. They are extremely useful throughout their life.

Discipline

Our world is one of instant gratification. it is as easy as pressing a button it is what we need. Everybody is multitasking, and frequently we don't really focus only on one thing simultaneously. Technology has made us lazy, as well as deprived us of essential life capabilities we need to be.

As you begin the path of calisthenics you've got a target or goals that you have in your mind about the things you would like to accomplish. You are aware that you require physical strength to accomplish the objectives you've set however, you'll also require determination and discipline to reach your goals.

It requires discipline to stay up even when you're tired or are failing to achieve a particular objective, even though you have tried your best. The exercise routine helps develop discipline by ensuring that you are determined to achieve your goals and achieve the goals that you set you.

Your mindset is developing to be successful, so too is your mental discipline as you take every move you make. The chain reaction occurs as you are focused on achieving your goals. In the end of your day, the commitment and the discipline that you've developed transfer to all aspects in your life. Your career, education and even your private life will all benefit from a the discipline of your mind.

Learn to Manage the Fear of Failure

Learning to do calisthenics helps you to handle the anxiety of not being able to do something. When you advance through your fitness routine there will be times when you'll fall short in the event that you lack determination to do your sets and the reps you set as your objective. It's a sign that you're failing when aren't able to smoothly complete a particular position and then you'll are prone to falling. This is a part the process of improving your the calisthenics.

Accepting that failure doesn't mean you're done and instead can be a process of learning will help you grow with your training as well as in different areas in your daily life. Apply this knowledge from calisthenics, and apply it to different areas in your daily life. There is no need to worry about failing. Take it as a challenge, clean off and attempt another time. Learning is not slipping up. Search for solutions to reach your objectives.

Self-Control

Training in Calisthenics teaches you to direct your body's movement. Learn the ability to lift as well as push it and move through a myriad of different methods that you were unable to accomplish prior to. The self-mastery philosophy that the calisthenics program is built on isn't new. A lot of ancient religious philosophical theories around the globe have their roots in this. Calisthenics-based self-mastery training goes beyond physical fitness in order to master the desires and emotions. Being able to manage your desires and emotions will benefit the entire course of your daily life. It influences how you manage circumstances, and also how you handle both good and as well bad triggers.

Self-Reliance

There are many ways their efforts to stay in their fitness and overall health. You can visit the gym, and utilize the rowing machine as well as the treadmill. Or they work out or utilize cross-training equipment. These people gain a lot from as well, and there's something to be gained from their techniques. However, the use of these machines and equipment, they depend on other tools in order to keep their fitness levels. Take away their equipment and all of a sudden, everything grinds to a abrupt halt.

When you do calisthenics, all you need to do is depend on yourself. It's not a problem without an exercise bike or treadmill. All you need is your body to reach your fitness targets. Self-reliance is learned without relying upon any external sources.

It's the same for your life all over the world. Consider how many times you've heard people say that they don't feel happy only if they have the money to buy costly products. Perhaps a person has mentioned at you about how they are unable to be confident in themselves until they are able to get the approval of their spouse or boss's approval. The problem is that they haven't learned to be independent.

It teaches you that just need your own efforts to attain healthy and fit as well as that you possess the tools to feel great. The only thing you must be able properly use the body and mind.

Physical Benefits

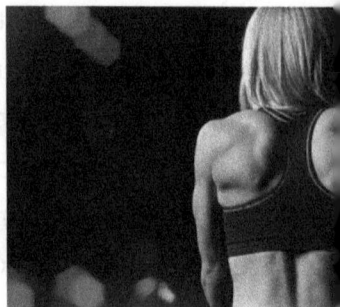

Regular calisthenics training has many health benefits for every fitness instructor. Health benefits can be in the short and long term, since some of them become significant over time. People who practice calisthenics have a greater quality of life when they age.

These benefits will make it worthwhile to do calisthenics even though it may sometimes be difficult:

Bone Density

The exercise program stimulates the growth of bone density. This is vitally important in order to avoid or lessen the chance of developing osteoporosis.

Chronic Conditions

The regular calisthenics exercise helps reduce or avoid a variety of chronic illnesses that can be dangerous, for example:

* Obesity

* Diabetes

* Arthritis

* Back back pain

* Heart disease

* Depression

* Hypertension

* High cholesterol

* Osteoporosis

Certain types of cancer

* Stroke

Cognitive Decline

Mental and physical discipline as a result of exercises can help prevent or lessen the negative effects of cognitive decline among older people.

Energy Levels

If you continue to work on calisthenics your strength will increase as well as your levels of energy are likely to increase noticeably.

Flexibility, Mobility, and Balance

The exercise helps maintain your balance and flexibility by increasing mobility. This is crucial when your body gets older so that you can remain independent and flexible.

Greater Stamina

The effects of Calisthenics are an ensuing chain reaction of more exercise, building strength as well as improved health and overall wellbeing, all of which help to increase strength and endurance.

Immune System

Fitness levels that are high as well as a healthy, balanced food plan help the immune system in its fight against illnesses.

Insomnia and Sleep

A boost in fitness and better psychological well-being promote better sleeping patterns, and significantly helps to reduce the issue of insomnia.

Muscle Strength and Tone

The increased protection for joints against injury is a result of an increase in muscular power.

Performance of Everyday Tasks

Through calisthenics, you develop functional strength and not only strength to lift the weights, or for putting your muscles to the test. Strong, lean muscles help in performing everyday tasks much simpler as they put less strain on joints and muscles.

Posture

Strengthening and flexibility of muscles helps improve posture.

Risk of Injury

The chance of injury diminishes as you progress, build muscle and strength increases.

Self-Esteem

If you adhere to a strict fitness program and notice the changes you're getting through the process of getting your body in shape It boosts confidence in yourself.

Sense of Wellbeing

The practice of resistance training can boost confidence and an image of your body that is positive. The increase in your perception of health and well-being boosts your state of mind.

Weight-Management and Muscle to Fat Ratio

Regular exercise will increase your muscles and help you burn off calories, even when you're sitting down. This helps make weight control simpler.

Mental and Emotional Wellbeing

Each human being desires to be content. Actually, happiness is a part of the human genome by way of a protein produced in the FAAH gene, which affects pleasure and pain. The most effective way to tell that calisthenics can improve the emotional and mental health of your family is to promote your experience with the Action for Happiness movement's GREAT Dream, also known as the 10 keys for a more joyful life. Calisthenics is directly linked to all of the 10 keys and is a great way to enhance your lifestyle and well-being.

Giving

It gives you the possibility to help other people through sharing your expertise and experience as you grow. Your time is an invaluable resource for helping other people through sharing what you've gained from your own experience and also to inspire other people to begin calisthenics.

Relating

The community of calisthenics is extremely intimate in comparison to other fitness and health-related communities. It is a non-competitive sport that promotes a spirit of openness and sharing that encourages friendship. This can be beneficial especially those who are new to the sport. They can connect with other people who share the same enthusiasm, and also find that lots of encouragement and moral support that is readily available.

Exercising

Our bodies weren't designed for a life of sedentary living. Our bodies were designed for moving. When we move more with, the greater our body releases endorphins. This is the hormone that makes us happy to put it in simple terms. Therefore, when you work out, your body will thank for your efforts by creating endorphins. These will make you feel better and provide you with a general sensation of happiness.

Appreciating

Calisthenics provides practitioners with two methods of experiencing satisfaction. One way is that it is possible go outside for your exercise. There is no requirement to workout within a particular location or building. The place you live in it is possible that you have the natural beauty close by and you can enjoy performing your reps and sets at a stunning green space. In any case it is possible to breathe fresh air and look around while doing it.

The other method is to practice mindful awareness. Calisthenics, like we mentioned earlier, is not just physically-based exercises. It affects your mind and sharpens your focus and helps you develop your mental discipline. By focusing on working out and striving to reach your goal it is not a waste of time worrying or stressing over aspects of your daily life that bother you or you are unable to effectively address.

Trying Out

The calisthenics training is an exercise that will always learn. You will always be working towards another goal to achieve, or perfecting your skills. Learning something new is infinite, since you are able to continue to explore new moves after you've mastered one.

Direction

Everyone needs goals they can anticipate throughout their lives or something that they can be striving for. It is a part of our behavior, and we're most content when we are able to clearly define our objectives of where we wish to be. Calisthenics provides a variety of goals that which you can accomplish with determination dedication, perseverance, and hard work.

Resilience

In the portion entitled Life Lessons in which we talked about how to manage the fear of failing. It is a mental health ability that calisthenics can teach you: being resilient, and having the capacity to come back from failure you've made a mistake. Physical challenges as well as the failures you face in training will help develop the ability to overcome the failures that occur in other areas of your daily life. When your body grows it will learn about you as well as the capacity you possess to conquer any obstacles on your path. It's a lesson that can be applied to the relationships you have with your family, work, your family and even your friends.

How to Balance Healthy Eating Socially

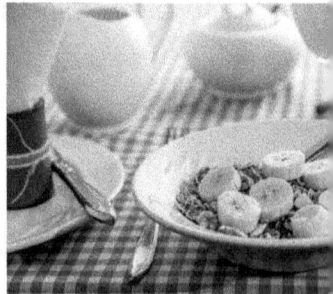

Eating out or socializing with friends can be stressful for people who is still in the early stages of the training for calisthenics. It is a lot of work for each step, but dining out with your friends or colleagues could take away many hours of effort. The result is a slowing down of your progress and could demotivate you which is not something anyone wants to do. This is why it's important to keep a few of suggestions to avoid those pitfalls of socializing or eating out, especially when you're dedicated to maintaining a healthy body and mind by doing exercises.

Check the Menu

Find out what's available on the menu before start of the meeting. So you don't have to select foods when you are exhausted or hungry or tired, as well as making poor choice of food on in the midst of your day.

Healthy Snack Before Arrival

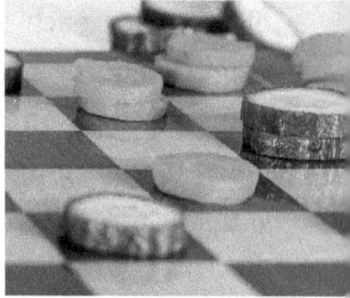

If we're hungry, it is common to consume more. When we dine out in any restaurant where the wait for food can be very long it could result in making the wrong choices about food and overeating. Consume a protein-rich, balanced snack, such as the yogurt or smoothie prior to when going to a eatery.

Water

A glass of water should be always on hand. Drink water prior to the start of your meal as well as throughout the meal, and drink the water in place of sweetened beverage. It will spare you lots of calories.

Check How Food is Prepped and Cooked

The method of preparation and cooked may have significant effect on the amount of calories and fat content in an item. The most popular buzz words include sauteed, crisp and pan-fried. Also, you can find crunchy and fried. These meals are generally more fat-rich as well as calories. Instead, search for steam poached, grilled or roasted dishes in the menu.

Order First

Our choices are often guided by the meal that others dining at tables order while dining out with a crowd. A great way to steer clear of the temptations and uncomfortable times is simply to place your order for meal before others can.

Double Up on Appetizers

Restaurants that specialize in serving massive portions which can lead to overeating. One way to prevent the problem is to choose two appetizers, instead of one massive main meal.

The food you eat will feel full without having the need for a huge intake of calories.

Mindful Eating

Mindful eating can change eating habits it is very beneficial when you are in a social setting where eating too much or poor eating habits are prevalent. The concept of mindful eating is to enjoy every flavor and smell in each bite as you pay attention to what sensations you are experiencing while you chew each item of food. As per findings of the study conducted in 2013 mindfulness-based eating is a way to develop control over eating, which prevents you from getting too hungry, as well as helps you make better eating choices in restaurants and social gatherings (Robinson and others.).

Eat Slowly and Chew Well

This method of coping with dining out is in conjunction with eating mindfully. Slowing down the pace of eating by consciously reducing your eating speed and attempting to chew every bite of food for X amount in a row, you body is given enough time to tell you that it is full prior to overeating.

Coffee Instead of Dessert

Avoid the temptation to eat dessert instead of ordering dessert and opt for a cup coffee instead. This can drastically cut down the calories you consume, as well as you'll actually reap the many positive health effects that coffee offers.

Request a Healthy Swap

After you have placed your order, ask for the substitution of high-calorie foods like fries, potatoes or pan-fried things. You can substitute these foods with veggies or salad.

Dressings and Sauces on the Side

It is a good idea to insist that sauces and dressings that you add to your food are served with the food. Dressings and sauces are known to be packed with calories and fats they can be controlled in the amount you consume easier when they are offered on the side.

Bread Basket

A bread and fruit basket served prior to dinner is an established practice in numerous eateries. If you're already starving at the time you get there and are hungry, you'll be likely to eat and then take your meal plan to the window. Instead, take your bread basket to stay away from the temptation.

Salad or Soup Starters

The study of 2007 showed you could reduce the calories consumed at an eating time by as high up to 20% if you begin by eating soup (Flood and Rolls 2007). It also proved that this is true regardless of the kind of soup you are using. It is an excellent method to cut down on calories as well as provide you with peace of mind regarding not having to interrupt your workout routine.

Share or Go Half-Portion

Individuals who adhere to portion control typically share meals together with a person sitting at the dining table. It's a great method to avoid overeating and also helps everyone. If you do not have anyone to share the meal with, you can ask the server for a portion of your meal. A majority of restaurants permit customers to request portions of half. If not inform them that you'd like to take portions of your meal and take it back home in a bag for your dog.

Alcohol, Mixers, and Sweetened Drinks

There is no requirement to be averse to alcohol in any form in your social gatherings. It's just a matter of thinking ahead and make decisions rationally. You can order a smaller glass of wine instead one large glass. You can also make sure you request an diet mixer when you're drinking mixer instead of spirits that is sweetened by sugar.

Drinking soft drinks may also add on calories while eating at restaurants. It's much better to sip water, non-sweetened beverages, or an unsweetened cup of tea.

Tomato-based in contrast to. Creamy Sauces

Beware of cheese sauces as well as sauces that contain cream. Instead, choose more nutritious options of tomato-based or vegetable-based sauces to make delicious tasting and lower calories.

Be Wary of Health Claims

It's not rare nowadays to find items that are listed on menus of restaurants as "sugar-free", "keto", "gluten-free", or "paleo". Be aware that"sugar-free" simply means that there's no sugar from cane in the food or dish. Most times, other types of sweeteners are being employed that are similar to or more calories as sugar.

This is also true of foods that are marketed as meeting the nutritional requirements of certain food groups, since certain foods are extremely rich in fats. Also, make sure you take the time to look at the menu, and don't fall into the trap of the sensationalism.

Chapter 11: The Fuel for Lean Living

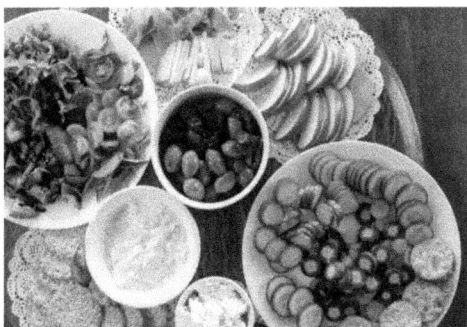

The process of building your body require an appropriate diet. In fact, wellbeing and health all around require a nutritious diet from the beginning. You must remember that what you consume influences your ability to exercise and also the results beginning before you begin the exercise program, throughout exercises, and even while relaxing.

The extent to which you'll need modify your eating habits will depend upon how well-balanced your diet is. If you're in an area of either over or eating too much and are unable to maintain the same healthy, regular diet, the first next step is to create an appropriate diet program. If you're not eating well it will be difficult to have enough motivation to work out and you may however, the outcomes will not be evident.

If you are looking to achieve an increase in the muscle mass, your diet is going to be required to follow the demands of your lifestyle. However the diet shouldn't be excessively demanding either. It's not easy to live without working out and eating as well as daily tasks and obstacles in life won't pay too much about the need to properly eat. The best way to ensure that you are eating a balanced, sustainable and practical eating plan if would like it to serve your long-term. If you're on a strict diet, it's difficult to maintain regardless of the apparent physical and mental health benefits. The process of implementing a healthy lifestyle is best accomplished step by step each day at a stretch, much the like starting to workout. We would like for you to succeed with your change. We recognize that not everyone can handle abrupt modifications.

Are you able to slip into a strict eating and fitness routine completely different from what you use to? It's unlikely. Fitness and health are acquired by taking one step at a regardless of the fact you'll start your day with a bang. day of exercise, you'll do 10 minutes for a mere ten minutes before giving away sweets. They're the kind of tiny changes that lead to massive changes in your life. For instance, one day you're performing ten squats, and then substituting regular pizza for the slim alternative. On the next day, you'll be doing ten pushups and ten lunges or eating the smoothie at breakfast instead of the usual sweet cereal. One year later in the future, and you'll be an entirely different person. Therefore, take your time with yourself and begin your new you.

In the beginning, adapting to a healthier diet plan to perform calisthenics requires regular adjustments to the size of your meals, food selections, and your eating habits. First, you have consider your health, body life style, goals, and lifestyle for determining the type of diet to follow. The first step is to calculate how much calories you will need for your workout days as well as the days you rest. Then, think about your fitness objective when creating a food strategy, such as:

* Muscle gain. If you've decided to use calisthenics in order to build muscle the daily calories you consume must be greater than the amount you consume. It is suggested that you increase your intake by 200-500 calories per every day food intake.

* Fat loss. If your aim is to shed fat, then you must create a calorie deficit of 200 to 500 calories per day in your eating habits. You still have ensure that your diet can support your regular physical exercise. Keep in mind that you'll be active throughout your off days. Eating in excess can slow the rate of metabolic rate.

General Diet Recommendations

Dietary guidelines for success in calisthenics should not be a problem. This article will provide some simple diet guidelines to adhere to.

Concentrate on the quality of your food. The guidelines for a healthy diet are usually vague and require lots of meats that are lean along with healthy carbs as well as vegetables. But, it is also important ensure that you are eating sufficient food in order to keep active. Do not fall into the mistake of cutting down on the amount of protein, carbohydrates, and fat to levels below the limit simply because you're trying to slim down. There is still a need for meats or rice as well as oats and oatmeal regardless of whether you're working to shed weight. However it is essential that your food choices be flexible and enjoyable too. There's no way to feel satisfied when you eat only healthy and cooked meals, but completely disregarding individual tastes. There is no reason not to cheat as well as enjoy some tasty foods that you normally like, as this can allow you to relax from being following a strict diet and make you feel that your efforts are worthwhile.

Take note of your appetite. Planning your meals based on the calorie chart may prevent your attention from the real hunger. There is a possibility of having an intense appetite and consume lots of food, but not be able to lose weight. It is also possible having a weak appetite, and consume a small amount of food however, be unable to shed weight. There is no way to be unavoidable. If it is the case that you are eating a lot but don't experience any weight gain, be attentive to whether you're eating enough protein as well as if you're training too hard. There's a chance that you require some rest in order to build hypertrophy. In contrast If you cut down on the amount of food you eat, and yet to lose pounds, it's likely that you're not eating enough. If that's the scenario, you could experience fatigue and slowing down but not feel an appetite as a result of stress. Also, review your workout and food regimen and see if the calorie content and the composition of your diet are in line with your daily calories. Sometimes, you aren't hungry enough to consume the calories you want. If you are struggling with your appetite it is possible to choose calories-rich foods that provide higher amounts of nutrients in smaller amounts. In addition it is possible to reduce the amount of fiber you consume, as grains and oats contain fibers that can reduce your appetite.

Take care when taking supplementation with protein. A diet well-adjusted with the exercise routine should provide enough protein to aid in building muscle and strength. It is best to only look into protein supplements when you are subject to certain diet restrictions, or have difficulty eating eggs, meat, or dairy.

Diet Plan Ideas

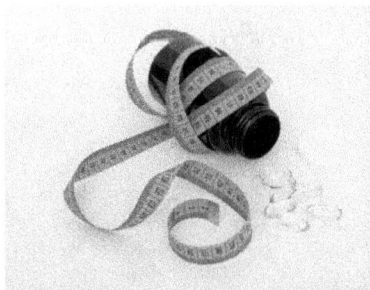

A healthy diet is essential to achieve optimal results in fitness when you do calisthenics, as well as in any other program of training. Inadequate nutritional balance could hamper your goals for fitness no matter how hard you work. If you're not accustomed to following the exact guidelines of a particular diet and aren't sure how to eat in order to get good results in calisthenics can be difficult. That's why this section will outline a healthy food plan to stick to when exercising calisthenics. The plan doesn't provide exact details of the foods you should eat and provide exact food amounts. Instead, it gives some general guidelines for creating an optimum diet, which is accompanied by regular physical activity. It is easy to alter portions and food options in accordance with your needs for the day.

For a balanced diet for exercise in calisthenics it isn't necessary to buy appliances for cooking or extravagant food items. Also, there's no reason to pay more for foods than you did previously or alter your routine in order to allow enough time cook. This plan for eating is flexible, allowing you to alter it according depending on your own personal tastes and personal preferences and also to meet your fitness objectives. The act of weighing the food you eat is among the most effective ways to modify portions and prevent under or over eating. Below are some basic tips for eating healthy when doing calisthenics.

• Eat all-natural foods. The best nutrients will be found by eating foods that are not processed. Foods that are processed don't just contain harmful chemical compounds. They're also refined for a greater time on the shelf, which means they're deprived of vital nutrients you require for growth of your strength and muscles. Instead, you should get macronutrients in natural meats, fish dairy, seafood eggs, and other seafood. Vegetables and fruits will give you the natural fibers, as well as carbs that come from sugar. Grains as well as root vegetables provide healthful carbs, too.

• Cut down on unhealthy foods. It is essential to cut out fast food, processed oils and junk food for a better chance of being healthier in general however, you should also be able to improve your the calisthenics. Additionally it is also important to eliminate white rice as well as all other items made with white flour. This includes pastries as well as pasta.

Do not limit your fruits or vegetables. There is no limit to the number of vegetables as you like, and they won't hinder the health of your body or results from exercise.

* Limit mealtimes. Don't spread meals throughout the day. You should instead eat in the eight hour time frame. This allows you to consume food when hungry, with no restrictions but keep you from becoming too hungry. If you're not starving it's less likely that you'll find yourself tempted by food items that aren't healthy. You'll instead eat meals with a higher calorie content as well as

consume fewer calories eating your food over the course of the day.

Be sure to supplement with caution. It is best to obtain all of your nutrients through your meals every day rather than supplements. If you're still feeling as though you'd benefit from supplementation You should consider these supplements with caution:

* Creatine. Creatine helps to heal from injuries, and aids in building muscles mass.

* Proteins. If you're worried that you don't have enough protein to help build muscle mass whether you're vegetarian or vegan supplementing your protein intake is a fantastic alternative to meat. Additionally, it can help recovering muscles injured in the event that you train too hard.

* The amino acids of the branched chain (also known as BCAA will help you increase your muscle mass and keep the gains you have made in the past.

* Vitamins. While you can easily consume enough vitamins from veggies and fruits, multivitamin supplements can aid in obtaining the nutrients difficult to get through food, such as Zinc B complex, zinc, as well as vitamins D, E D as well as C.

In order to understand how you can consume a healthy diet while doing calisthenics, be able to figure the macronutrients you consume in your daily food plan. Carbs, fats as well as protein need a proper amount in your diet for the best performance results. Learn how to obtain enough healthy macronutrients

* Carbohydrates. It is important to eat complex carbohydrates. They won't increase blood sugar levels and trigger excessive blood glucose to build up in the fat cells. Complex carbs are found in the fruits and vegetables you eat Whole grains, nuts as well as seeds. The fiber in fruits and vegetables can also be broken down into carbohydrates after consumption.

* Fats. Apart from the fats that are naturally present in dairy products, meat as well as nuts and seeds It is also recommended to use healthy fats in cooking. A good choice is olive oil that is extra virgin and coconut oil. The saturated fats are present in the meats as well as tropical plants such as coconuts. Unsaturated fats can be found in the form of nuts, fish and even vegetables. Reduce your consumption of saturated fats by consuming low-fat meats because our bodies are able to create them by themselves. But essential fatty acids such as omega 3, and 6, need to be sourced via eating habits. That's why it's recommended to consume at minimum 2 servings of fish per weekly, and also to make use of small amounts of Extra virgin olive oil in cooking. But even these fats may cause obesity in large quantities.

* Proteins. Proteins are the building blocks of your nails, muscles, hair and ligaments and help to maintain your body's movement. These are amino acids which are the building blocks of muscles. If you are looking for

sources of nutritious protein, try healthy fish and lean meats, as well as dairy that is lean, eggs and mushrooms as well as legumes and legumes. The foods mentioned above can be consumed in huge quantities without contributing to weight gain.

* Micronutrients. The last but certainly not least is the minerals and vitamins present in both vegetables and fruits. Vitamins are essential to help support the body's biological functions as well as in the context of fitness, they help ensure that you have solid and secure movements. A deficiency of vitamins often impacts the metabolism of your body, performance levels and appearance.

Eating Tips and Meal Ideas

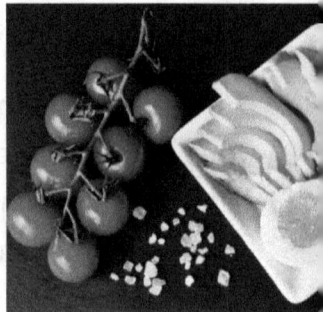

In the past, we've offered the general advice on eating right while doing calisthenics. In this part we've included a few of ideas for food options from the morning to evening, for you to get an idea of how your typical daily meal ought to appear in.

Breakfast

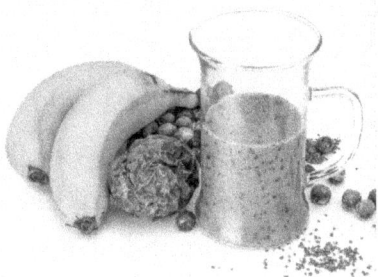

Oatmeal and Fruit

Ingredients:

* 1 cup whole Oats

1 cup regular, almond or coconut milk.

* 1 cup berries

* up to 1 cup of crushed nuts

Instructions:

It is essential to have a nutritious breakfast to fuel you up for the day, and oatmeal with any berries you want (strawberries blueberries, strawberries, or mixed berries) along with fruit like mangoes, bananas and oranges, are an ideal choice. A bowl with one serving is usually an adequate amount regardless of age or gender However, you may alter the breakfast you eat to increase or decrease calories if you need to. If, for instance, you're looking to eat a lighter breakfast, opt for almond or coconut milk in place of regular or limit your fruit consumption. However should you wish to enhance the calorific content for the meal it is possible to increase the amount to up to one cups of nuts. Remember that nuts contain a lot of calories and can add as much as 200 calories in a dinner. Fruits and berries are essential in providing sufficient sugar however in a safe manner and, of course, in order to provide fiber and support the digestive system.

Fruit Salad

Ingredients:

* Fruits that have been chopped (bananas and avocados or oranges, pineapple, raspberries, or strawberries)

* 1 tbsp. raw honey

* 1 tbsp. lemon juice

Instructions:

If you'd prefer a less hefty breakfast, it is possible to consume as many bananas, oranges, avocados, berries, avocados or apples as you like. How to consume enough fruit is to chew it and chew slowly. limit your consumption to at which you feel satisfied.

Breakfast Tortilla

Ingredients:

One whole wheat tortilla

Topping with fruit:

* 1 cup of chopped fruit

* 1 tbsp. almond or peanut butter

* One cup or more of crushed nuts

For vegetable topping:

* Cut vegetables (tomatoes and spinach or onions)

* A drop of olive oil

* 1 tbsp. lemon juice

* A teaspoon of salt

* A little bit of pepper

* 1 teaspoon of every spice that you like (parsley or basil, etc.)

* 1 slice cheddar cheese

* Greek yogurt

Instructions:

Whole wheat tortillas are an ideal breakfast alternative regardless of gender or fitness targets. Breakfast will be a light meal if you fill your tortilla with fruit (berries as well as bananas and avocados) or other vegetables (sliced tomatoes leaves, green leafy vegetables and cucumbers, olives, for example.). If you'd like to enhance calories in your meal, include an almond or peanut butter when you prefer fruits. You can also you can add a cup Greek yogurt with the wrap of vegetables. This can add fat to the food if you're training in a higher-volume. Alternately, you could make substitutions for some of the ingredients by adding cheddar cheese or the kale in order to enhance your breakfast with more healthy calories.

Green smoothie

Ingredients:

* 1 handful spinach

One apple

* 1 handful of leaves from kale

* One banana

* 1 tbsp. lemon juice

1 cup almond or coconut milk.

* Water, as necessary

Instructions:

There is a lot of debate about whether or not a fruit smoothie is the most nutritious breakfast choice. You can decide your choice if you include enough carbohydrates into the smoothie. It is possible to put any green vegetables you enjoy in a blender, however the apple with a few handfuls of spinach leaves, a bit of lemon juice, kale and the addition of a banana is an excellent choice. If you find your smoothie to be lacking in nutrients, include fruit like either a full or half banana or some berries, for flavor, vitamins as well as calories. Do you have a lack of carbohydrates? You can add up to one cup of whole oats or if you're performing intensive training, include a cup of coconut milk or almonds. It's clear that there are numerous healthy methods to boost or calculate the calorific content of your beverage The choice is entirely yours!

Lunch and Dinner

The great thing about healthy food is its flexibility. The meals of lunch and dinner mix the flavors of vegetables, meats, herbs and spices which can be consumed throughout the day as well as at night. To make it easier We suggest cooking an entire meal, and then eating one portion for lunch as well as a second serving for dinner. In contrast in the event that you don't wish to have the same food every day, then you could prepare a few meals beforehand. Lunchtime meals need to be balanced with carbohydrates and protein. The reason for this is that the food items with the highest macronutrients include a lot of fat. All together can raise blood sugar levels and cause the food to become too excessively heavy.

Always remember to use only organic processed, and natural foods. Here are a few suggestions for balanced, healthy food that is satisfying and balanced:

Fish and vegetables

Ingredients:

* 1 salmon - 2 salmon or other seafood of your choice (a portion of the size of a palm)

2. Cups or more of chopped broccoli, kale, cauliflower and zucchini. and eggplant

* 1 tbsp. extra olive oil

* 1 tbsp. lemon juice

* 1/2 tbsp. chopped parsley

* 1 teaspoon dill

* 1 TSP basil

* A teaspoon of salt

* A little bit of pepper

Instructions:

The process of cooking fish shouldn't be difficult. If you do not like cooking much then you could grill a small piece of fish and boil the fish. If you'd like to enhance the flavour however it is easy to top the salmon with extra virgin olive oil, and then sprinkle it with herbs, including powdered onion and parsley or dill. In this recipe, cook a portion of salmon and a vegetable-based side-dish that is consisting of chopped and sauteed the following vegetables: broccoli, spinach and zucchini. You can also add cauliflower, cauliflower and eggplant. Don't forget your avocado! The avocado can be served alongside your veggies if you are a fan of this type of blend and also serve it for dessert.

Vegetables and meat

Ingredients:

* 1 - 2 chicken breasts

* 2 cups or more chopped broccoli, kale, cauliflower, spinach, paprika and zucchini

Extra Virgin Olive Oil

* A teaspoon of salt

* A little bit of pepper

* 1 cup vegetable stock

* 1/2 tbsp. chopped parsley

* 1/2 tsp of basil

* 1/2 tsp dill

* 1/2 tsp ginger

Instructions:

This same method for making an energizing, protein-rich meal is also used for cooking for meat. All you require is an ounce of meat that you cook or grill according to your preference! Be sure to use only the maximum amount of olive oil extra-virgin.

As a side dish it is possible to stir fry chops of sweet potatoes (up up to 2 cups) and chop vegetables from your choice all in one (e.g. broccoli, kale as well as spinach) then stir fry along with a small amount of water or even a container of stock for vegetables.

Are you looking to add some spice? Include chopped onion, parsley and basil sprinkle with a teaspoon of lime or lemon juice.

Beans/Legumes Stir Fry Vegetables

Ingredients:

* 2 cups of quinoa, brown rice, beans

* 2 cups of chopped veggies of your choice

* 1 onion sliced

* 1 tbsp. extra olive oil

* A teaspoon of salt

* A small amount of pepper

1 cup of vegetable or chicken stock

Instructions:

And now, hold your breath. Do you really need every day eat a pound of meat for a ripped body? No one really is, even nutritional experts. In this option for meals it is recommended to substitute an ounce of meat and up to 2 cups of quinoa or beans. Less-fat meals typically have cups, whereas those looking to build muscles and weight usually opt with two cups or two smaller cans.

First, boil your legumes for 30 minutes. You'll have them ready to consume although they're not particularly tasty. Make sure you have a pan and one teaspoon of olive oil. Incorporate chopped onions, and allow to simmer for a few minutes before adding half cup of water or vegetable broth. In order to increase the amount of calories in lean it is possible to use chicken stock. Add your rice or quinoa to mix it all in and allow to simmer for 5 minutes. The meal is almost done The only thing you'll need to do is include up to 2 cups of vegetables finely chopped Add more broth or water (up to the size of a glass) then let it simmer for at least ten minutes. Enjoy!

In this section you've been taught how to cook the basic food to help you maintain fitness and support the growth of your muscles. What about pre- and post-workout meals? In the next section we'll discuss the benefits of smoothies for health as well as how you can make smoothies quickly and efficiently.

Chapter 12: Beginning by Using Smoothies

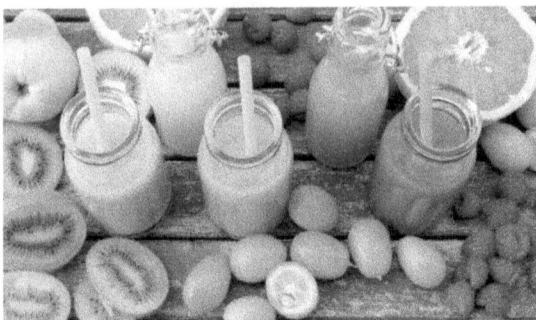

Smoothies aren't just intended for weightlifters, bodybuilders or dedicated gym-goers. Smoothies taste great as well as a great source of protein at the time you're in need regardless of whether you are using them used for breakfast, in the post-workout period or even as a great snack. The selection of flavors you can create is endless and you are able to alter the sweetness level and add flavorings according to your own personal preferences.

An important note on protein powders: note that these supplements do not have the status of being FDA controlled. Thus, the huge variety of brands and options offered on the market could differ greatly from one another. Research to determine which protein powder will best suit your needs.

There are many methods to get ready for smoothies that can save the time and effort. Most people it is a busy life so any way to reduce the time spent preparing meals is an enormous benefit.

Frozen Fruit vs. Fresh

In the absence of a consistent availability of fresh fruits and items available throughout the day The first option is to begin building up the stocks of frozen fruits. There are containers for frozen fruits in the majority of supermarkets and you could also create your own. It's an excellent idea to keep your most-loved fruit in single servings, in glass jars, plastic containers or ziplock bags for the freezer. So, you'll be able to take a container out and create a smoothie without needing to consider portions.

Make-Ahead Smoothie Packs

The frozen containers of fruit one step further and prepare your smoothies in advance. This can prove extremely helpful to every household that has multiple people who drink smoothies. It is also a cost-effective option when purchasing fruits and vegetables in bulk.

Cleanse and wash all veggies and fruits. Next, you need to measure every ingredient for the particular smoothie you wish to create and put all the ingredients into single smoothie containers in the freezer. These smoothie packs may be stored in the refrigerator to be used over the course of a few days.

This is by far the most efficient method you could prepare a smoothie because all you need to do is include the liquid since all of the vegetables and fruits were prepared.

Quick Fix Remedies

Sometimes, we'll have smoothies that are either too sweet or too thick or doesn't have the level of tartness you like. Below are some easy solutions to assist in the event of a problem. Combine the ingredients in order to change the flavor or thickness. Then, blend for an additional 10-20 seconds so that everything is incorporated.

To make it too thick, add some milk, juice, or water and mix. Continue blending if the mix remains too heavy.

To make it too thin, add any of the ingredients listed below to thicken the mix:

* Banana

* Strawberries

* Frozen yogurt

* Extra ice

* Chia seeds

* Oats that are raw

* Protein powder

* Xanthan gum

* Avocado

* Silken tofu

* Nut butter

The bitter taste of mature greens generally have a bitter flavor The best method to mitigate the bitterness is by using young greens since they possess a milder flavor. It is possible to add one of these ingredients to reduce bitterness of the dish:

* Bananas are a good choice due to their neutralizing effect against bitter flavor

* Strawberries sweeten smoothies made with greens exceptionally well.

* Vanilla extract or vanilla bean

* Agave

* Cocoa powder, also known as unsweetened cocoa powder

Too sweet: add concentrated frozen lemonade, or freshly squeezed lemon juice

Insufficiently sweet Incorporate sweeteners and other ingredients that make the smoothie sweeter by adding small pieces each time and not over-sweeten it. Ingredients are:

* Watermelon instead of water

* Agave syrup, honey, sugar or maple syrup

* Stevia, or any artificial sweetener of your personal preference

* Grapes

* Dates

If you aren't sure if it is creamy enough, try one of the ingredients listed on this list for help in creating an even more creamy taste.

* Avocado

* Ice cream

* Vanilla yogurt

* Frozen yogurt

Substitutions

Many smoothie recipes advise users to only use certain natural ingredients. It is possible to substituting every ingredient in a recipe for smoothies by using a different ingredient that is more suitable to your individual needs and preferences. In addition, using plants-based ingredients rather than animal-based ingredients makes recipes vegetarian and vegan.

These ingredients as well as substitutes are able in the preparation of delicious protein shakes that delight everyone.

* Dairy milk

* Soy milk

* Hemp milk

* Almond milk

* Oat milk

* Cashew milk

* Rice milk

* Sorghum milk

* Coconut milk

* Flax milk

* Nuts

* Sunflower seeds, also known as the sunflower butter that is made of seeds (sun butter)

* Pumpkin seeds (pepitas)

* Tahini

* Flax seeds

* Chia seeds

* Hemp seeds

* Sugar honey

* Maple syrup

* Rice syrup made from brown rice

* Agave nectar

* Malt barley syrup

* Sorghum syrup

* Stevia or an Artificial sweetener or option

* Dates

* Grapes

* Whole eggs

* Ener-G eggs purchased from stores

* 1 tbsp. agar flakes

* 1 tbsp. applesauce

* 1 banana mashed

* 1/4 cup silken tofu

* 1/4 cup coconut yogurt

* 1 tbsp. ground flax seeds or Chia seeds simmered for 2 mins in 3 tablespoons. of water (or allowed to cool in the refrigerator for 15 minutes)

* Egg whites and aquafaba

* Any of the substitutions mentioned for whole eggs

* Spinach, bok choy

* Kale

* Radish greens

* Parsley

* Dandelion greens

* Arugula

* Turnip greens

* Celery

* Celery greens

* Collard greens

* Swiss Chard

* Mustard greens

* Romaine lettuce

* Broccoli

* Beet greens

* Broccoli * rabe (rapini)

* Carrot greens

* Dairy yogurt

* Protein powder

* Coconut cream

* Yogurt made with almond milk

* Chia seeds

* Ripe avocado

Blending Tips and Tricks

It is our goal to make the most delicious smoothies with the least amount of duration of time. Therefore, these tips will be helpful to ease the process and make the process more efficient.

There are a variety of electronic stand blender with a high-speed motor, or even a jug with an immersion blender to create smoothies. The main difference between these two types of blenders is that the stand blender is more powerful. It allows the stand-mixer to blend more effectively ingredients, such as vegetables that are cruciferous, frozen food items, as well as frozen ingredients, and ice cubes.

The blender should be loaded with your desired ingredients according to the order as follows:

Then, you pour in the liquid.

Add small and soft ingredients.

Put any greens over the.

Put frozen fruits and vegetables on top of the leaves.

Finally, you can include any ice cubes that you'd like to put in.

One of the best tools to buy if you own a stand-mixer but doesn't come with it as an option such as an ice-cream tamper for your blender. It is utilized to get rid of any air pockets that may exist in the blender's jug as well as to force the mix into the blender's blades.

Do your best, but be careful not to overmix ingredients. Keep in mind that the motor and blades will begin to heat quickly and begin melting the ingredients that are frozen. Blend for 30-45 seconds, and then repeat as needed.

In the event of the ingredient that are used in a particular smoothie You may need stop the blender and scrub the sides of it clean before giving it a quick whirlwind.

If you're using coconut, other varieties of seeds, oatmeal, or nuts in whole form, include them in the blender along with the liquid. Blend these ingredients along with the liquid until you've got an extremely smooth paste. This should take about 30 minutes. After that, add the rest of the ingredients.

If you don't have the high-speed blender, it is better when you grated vegetables like beets, zucchini and carrots prior to adding them into the blender's container.

Smoothie Recipes

Orange and Mango Recovery Smoothie

This drink is sweet it is infused with turmeric which provides anti-inflammatory qualities that help in recovering. The recipe is vegan, is free of added sugar as well as being high in antioxidants and vitamin C. Protein's primary source is powdered protein.

5. Minutes

The Total Time is 5 minutes

Serving Size: 1

Ingredients

1. Cup almond milk unsweetened or any other dairy products of your preference

1. Cup mango block that are frozen

1. 1 scoop (2 heaping tablcspoons.) Vanilla protein powder made from vegans, vanilla

1 banana Frozen

* 1/2 tsp of turmeric (optional in order to enhance the anti-inflammatory qualities)

1. 1 orange from the naval frozen, peeled and then cut into pieces

* 1/2 tsp vanilla extract or essence

* 1 tbsp. hemp seeds (optional)

Directions

Mix all of the ingredients in a blender with high speed.

Blend until smooth.

Pour it into a glass and drink the beverage.

Green Breakfast Protein Smoothie

It's a great breakfast smoothie packed with vitamins and minerals and healthful fats from pumpkin seeds and hemp hearts. Protein powder can be added to give you additional protein.

In order to make this drink non-nut, you can substitute the almond milk with oatmeal hemp, coconut, hemp rice or soymilk.

5. mins

Total Time: 5 Minutes

Serving Dimension 2 cups (1 big serving)

Ingredients

* 1 fresh frozen banana (can be substituted for 2/3 cups peach chunks)

*1 cup almond milk without sweetener, or substitute it for milk of your preference

* 1/2 cup frozen mango chunks

* 2 large chunks of baby spinach or kale that has been destemmed

* 2 tbsp. hemp heart (hemp seeds which are removed from the hull)

* 1/4 cup pepitas (pumpkin seeds)

1. 1/2-1 scoop (1-2 heaped tablespoons.) protein powder, vanilla flavor

* 1/4 cup of water (optional)

Directions

Put all the ingredients in the blender container and blend until the pepitas have been completely integrated and soft.

It's a huge portion which means you could take it as breakfast or break it up into two smaller portions, and then use the other half for an early-morning snack.

Cinnamon, Oats, and Apple

If you're an oatmeal fan then this is the perfect smoothie. It's great for breakfast, morning snack, or even lunch. Oats are a slow discharge of energy which can keep you going for hours. almond butter and oats provide the majority of your protein. It is also possible to incorporate hemp hearts to boost your consumption of protein. The hemp doesn't alter the taste of your smoothie. If you want to get a substantial boost of protein it is possible to include vanilla protein powder also.

5. Minutes

The Total Time is 5 minutes

Serving Size: 1 large portion

Ingredients

* 1 cup oats in a roll

* 1 medium-sized to small-sized apple

* 1/2 tsp ground nutsmeg

* 1 1/2 tsp cinnamon powder

* 1 cup coconut milk unsweetened, not sweetened

* 1 tbsp. almond butter

* 2 tbsp. hemp heart (optional)

1. 1 scoop (2 heaping tablespoons.) Vanilla Protein powder (optional)

* 1 cup of water cold

* 3-4 cubes of ice

Directions

Add the water and oatmeal into the blender container and then pulse it a couple of times.

Place the blender jug in the refrigerator for about 2 minutes, to allow the oats time for softening.

Add the remainder of ingredients into the blender and mix for approximately 30 seconds until the mix is well-mixed.

* Pour the drink into a large glass, then garnish with cinnamon and nutmeg as garnish.

* Enjoy immediately.

Acai Berry and Mint

The smoothie can be enjoyed practically anytime of the day to have breakfast, after a workout for a post-workout snack, or a breakfast snack. Using protein powders that are unflavored lets the fruit and mint flavors to be kept in the forefront. The addition of ground seeds creates an extra thick drink with an excellent protein source. The tart cherry and mango puree as well as the acai berry purée is available in single serving containers, or utilize frozen fruit that you have in your freezer.

The Prep time is 5 mins

The Total Time is 5 minutes

Serving Size 1 large

Ingredients

* 1 frozen banana, sliced

* 1 orange fresh (Cara Care, Valencia, and Navel oranges are good)

1/2 cup mango frozen (or 1 packet of tart cherries and mango puree frozen (3.5 1 oz.)

* 3.5 oz. of frozen Acai fruit, or one box of frozen Acai puree (3.5 OZ.)

* 1 tbsp. flax seeds crushed

* 1 tbsp. chia seeds, ground

*1 scoop (2 heaping tablespoons.) protein powder that is unflavored

* 2 tbsp. hemp seeds crushed

* 1 cup coconut milk unsweetened, not sweetened

* 4-5 mint leaves, fresh

Directions

Add all of the ingredients in the blender and mix until it's soft.

Pour the contents into the glass of a large size and serve right away, when it is cold.

Avocado and Matcha along with Vanilla

This drink is refreshing, and matcha, that is a type made from powdered green tea offers many health benefits. The recipe is gluten and soy-free. This smoothie can be made by using only the essential ingredients, or include other ingredients depending on what you prefer.

5. Minutes

The Total Time is 5 minutes

Serving Size: 1

Ingredients

1. 1 Cup almond milk or a milk of your choice

* 1/2 avocado

1 tsp of matcha powder (start at half a teaspoon as it's potent)

*1 scoop (2 heaping tablespoons.) protein powder, vanilla (rice or pea protein works well)

* 2 - 4 ice cubes

* 1/2 cup of frozen fruits of your choice (optional)

* 2 tbsp. Flax seeds, chia seeds or even pepitas (optional)

* A couple of dates for sweets (optional)

* 2 to 3 tbsp maple syrup for added sweet (optional)

Directions

All the ingredients in the blender, and blend until the mixture is smooth.

* Serve promptly.

Cranberry, Banana, and Peanut Butter

They are an excellent addition to every smoothie as they are packed with antioxidants and vitamins as well as anti-inflammatory qualities in addition. They are both sweet, and it is recommended to make use of unsweetened fruits and vegetables. If you'd like for it to be sweeter make use of peanut butter that has added sugar and then add an additional sweeteners to the smoothie for example, maple syrup or honey. syrup. The protein source of this smoothie is peanut butter, as well as protein powder. This provides approximately 1.2 2 oz. of protein.

The Prep time is 5 mins

Total Time: 5 Minutes

Serving Dimension: 1 large portion

Ingredients

* 1 large frozen banana, sliced

1 cup of coconut milk non-sweetened, or the milk of one's own

* 2 tbsp. of peanut butter without sweetener

1. 1/4 cup dried cranberries not sweetened or sweetened with juice of fruit only

* 2 heaping Tbsp. Unflavored protein powder

* 1 1/2 tbsp. ground Chia seeds

* 1 tbsp. ground hemp seeds

* 3-4 cubes of ice

* Shredded coconut is an alternative topping

* Cacao nibs for an option for topping

Directions

* Crush the hemp seeds and the chia seeds with an espresso grinder prior to adding the mixture of smoothies.

* Add the milk along with ground seeds in the blender. Pulse until the mixture is well-mixed.

Mix all remaining ingredients to the blender and blend until the mix is completely well-mixed.

* Pour smoothies into an enormous glass. Add any optional toppings you wish to add then take a sip and enjoy.

Quinoa made with Strawberry and Banana

Quinoa is extremely high in protein. It also contains all the nine vital amino acids your body needs. It is high in fiber and magnesium. Chia seeds are the most abundant sources of plant-based Omega 3, and provide the highest amount of Omega 3 than salmon. Wheat germ is a great source of Vitamin B and fiber to the beverage to provide an all-round vitamin and protein smoothie that can be enjoyed at any time in the day. Quinoa can be cooked ahead of time, and then portion it into small portions, and then freeze it for later use to cut down on the time and energy.

Timing of Prep: 6 Minutes

The Total Time is 6 Minutes

Serving Size 2 cups (4 cups)

Ingredients

* 1/2 cup cooked quinoa, cooled down

* 1 banana that is ripe, huge

* 2 tbsp. honey

* 6 oz Greek yogurt, vanilla

* 1 tbsp. wheat germ

* 1 tbsp. chia seeds

2 cups of frozen strawberries (if you are using fresh strawberries then freeze them before freezing)

* 1/2 cup almond milk vanilla flavor (or the milk of your choice)

* 1 teaspoon the xanthan gum (optional in case you'd want a thicker, more smoky smoothie)

* 1 cup cubes of ice

Directions

All the ingredients in the blender and mix for approximately 45 seconds until the mix is silky smooth.

Pour the mixture into two glasses large enough to serve right away.

Banana, Peach, and Honey

The smoothie is popular among kids and adults alike as a breakfast option or snack. Protein's main ingredient can be found in cottage cheese. Protein powder that is unflavored can be added to the recipe for an additional powerful protein booster. This recipe yields 2 huge smoothies or three medium one.

5. Minutes

The Total Time is 5 minutes

Serving Size 2 smoothies

Ingredients

2. 1/2 cup of peach pieces in a freezer

* 1 banana that is ripe and fresh, or frozen

1 cup milk (full cream, low-fat or fat-free) may be substituted for any other plant-based milk

* 1 cup cottage cheese that is cultured, but preferably

* 2 tbsp. honey (more than less, may be utilized as per your individual preferences)

Directions

All ingredients in the blender. Blend until you achieve the consistency of a fine powder.

* Pour the mixture into two large glasses, and serve.

Pineapple and Raspberries

The recipe makes 3 cups for one serving. If you feel that this recipe is excessive, you could choose to add simple cottage cheese, and some milk. You can then make two portions. Protein comes from protein powder along with the cottage cheese is an option if you want to add it.

The Prep time is 5 Minutes

Total Time: 5 Minutes

Serving size: One huge portion (3 cups)

Ingredients

* 12 cup frozen, or fresh raspberries

* 1 cup frozen pineapple chunks

1 cup of coconut milk that is unsweetened

* 1/2 teaspoon Stevia (optional) or honey (optional)

* 2 tbsp. Protein powder with vanilla flavor of your preference

* 1/2 cup ice

* 1 cup plain cultured cottage cheese (optional additional)

* 1/4 cup additional coconut milk (optional additional if making cottage cheese)

Shredded coconut that is unsweetened for a garnish

Directions

All the ingredients in the bowl in a blender with a high speed and blend until the mix becomes thick and smooth consistency.

* Pour the mixture into a big glass, or two glasses of medium size.

Sprinkle with coconut shredded or other toppings you like and serve.

Cantaloupe and Ginger Smoothie

This recipe is focused primarily on cantaloupe rather than the typical assortment of fruits and seeds, nuts, and other vegetables used in the majority of smoothies. Protein is the main ingredient for this smoothie is Greek yogurt as well as cottage cheese. Protein powder that is unflavored can be used if you want to boost the protein content of your daily diet.

It is possible to transform this drink into a bowl of smoothies by adding an additional 1/2 cups of Greek yogurt. You can also top it off with coconut toasted, chopped Kiwi fruits, and Chia seeds.

7. mins

The Total Time is 7 mins

Serving Size Serving Size: 2 cups (2 portions of one cup or 1 big serving)

Ingredients

* * 2 1/2 cups peeled cantaloupe cut into pieces

* 1 cup Greek yogurt, plain

* 1/2 cup of cultured cottage cheese

1 Tbsp fresh ginger peeled and grated

* 1/2 tsp lime zest, finely grated

* 1 scoop (1 heaping tablespoon.) Unflavored protein powder (optional)

* 2 Tbsp maple syrup or honey

Directions

Add all of the ingredients in a blender and mix for around 30-60 seconds or until the mixture becomes soft and smooth.

- Serve right away as one big smoothie or two cups of one cup each.